PAIN
Creative Approaches to
Effective Management

Also by Eileen M. Mann and Eloise C.J. Carr:

Partnering Patients to Manage Pain After Surgery (1998) (video and 48-page
  booklet) Institute of Health and Community Studies, Bournemouth University.
Pain Management (2006) Oxford, Blackwell Publishing.

Pain

CREATIVE APPROACHES TO EFFECTIVE MANAGEMENT

Second Edition

Eileen M. Mann
Eloise C.J. Carr

palgrave
macmillan

First edition published 2000
Reprinted six times
Second edition published 2009 by
PALGRAVE MACMILLAN

Palgrave Macmillan in the UK is an imprint of Macmillan Publishers Limited, registered in England, company number 785998, of Houndmills, Basingstoke, Hampshire RG21 6XS.

Palgrave Macmillan in the US is a division of St Martin's Press LLC, 175 Fifth Avenue, New York, NY 10010.

Palgrave Macmillan is the global academic imprint of the above companies and has companies and representatives throughout the world.

Palgrave® and Macmillan® are registered trademarks in the United States, the United Kingdom, Europe and other countries.

ISBN-13: 978–0–230–20899–5
ISBN-10: 0–230–20899–1

This book is printed on paper suitable for recycling and made from fully managed and sustained forest sources. Logging, pulping and manufacturing processes are expected to conform to the environmental regulations of the country of origin.

A catalogue record for this book is available from the British Library.

10 9 8 7 6 5 4 3 2 1
18 17 16 15 14 13 12 11 10 09

Printed and bound in China

Contents

List of Figures		vii
List of Tables		viii
Foreword		ix
Preface		xi
Acknowledgements		xii
Introduction		xiii

1   The Multidimensional Nature of Pain   1
Background   2
Why has pain been so misunderstood?   2
An introduction to neurophysiology   6
Gate control theory   10
The psychosocial impact of pain   16
Neuromatrix theory   21
Conclusion   23
Multiple choice test   24

2   Assessing Pain   26
Background   27
Why assess pain?   27
When to assess pain   29
How to assess pain   29
Nurse factors affecting the assessment of pain   32
Patient factors affecting the assessment of pain   32
Pain assessment tools   35
Changing practice: introducing a pain assessment tool   50
Conclusion   51
Multiple choice test   52

3   Recognising the Barriers to Effective Pain Relief   55
Background   56
Healthcare professionals   56
Improving practice   59
Patient barriers to effective pain management   63
Organisational aspects   67
Barriers to effective pain management in the clinical area   68
Conclusion   72
Multiple choice test   73

4   Managing Acute Pain   76
Background   77

The patients' perspective: experiencing acute pain 78
Acute pain services 80
Pharmacological approaches to pain management 86
Non-pharmacological approaches to acute pain management 103
Conclusion 107
Multiple choice test 109

5 **Managing Chronic Pain** **112**
Background 113
What is chronic non-malignant or persistent pain? 114
The patient's perspective: experiencing chronic pain 117
Managing chronic pain 119
Pharmacological approaches to pain management 120
Non-pharmacological strategies for managing chronic pain 125
Physical techniques for managing pain 126
Psychological interventions 130
Herbs and supplements 133
Other considerations when managing pain 134
Professional collaboration in pain management 136
Conclusion 138
Multiple choice test 139

6 **Managing Pain in Vulnerable Patients** **142**
Background 143
Defining the barriers 145
Pain in the older person 146
Pain management in the cognitively impaired older person 149
Learning disability and brain-injured patients 155
Neonates and preverbal children 156
Ethnic minorities 164
Conclusion 167
Multiple choice test 168

7 **Nursing Patients with Challenging Pain** **171**
Background 172
Pain following a serious burn 173
Pain in the patient with a spinal injury 177
Pain in patients with sickle-cell disease 180
Mood disorder and pain 183
Substance misuse 187
Intractable pain and secondary gain/loss 192
Conclusion 197
Multiple choice test 197

Glossary 201
References 208
Index 224

List of Figures

1.1 The synaptic activity of A delta fibres in the spinal cord   7
1.2 The synaptic activity of C fibres in the spinal cord   9
1.3 Activity of A beta fibres in the spinal cord   10
1.4 Touch, pinprick and burning sensations transmitted to the brain via the
     dorsal horn of the spinal cord   10
1.5 Gate control theory: how a gate may be opened or closed   11
1.6 Response to the chemical cascade caused by tissue damage   14
1.7 Receptor activity   17

2.1 Visual analogue scale   35
2.2 Examples of pain scales   36
2.3 London Hospital pain observation chart   36
2.4 Short-form McGill Pain Questionnaire   37
2.5 The Brief Pain Inventory   40
2.6 The LANSS Pain Scale   42
2.7 Chart for recording acute pain intensity   44
2.8 Acute pain assessment chart   45
2.9 Epidural pain assessment and monitoring chart   49

4.1 An example of a sticky label covering a range of analgesia to treat
     acute pain   83
4.2 Algorithm for administration of intravenous opioids   84
4.3 Entonox delivery apparatus   97
4.4 The WHO pain ladder   99
4.5 Location of needle in epidural space   102
4.6 A TENS machine attached to a patient's belt with electrodes on
     the body   107

6.1 Example of preprinted analgesia prescription for acute pain in children   161

7.1 Physical and psychological influences on pain   173

List of Tables

1.1	Endogenous opioids and commonly administered opioids	15
1.2	Activity of opioids at the three receptor sites	16
4.1	Incidence of chronic pain after surgery	77
4.2	Popular NSAIDs divided into their chemically related groups	88
6.1	Common causes of pain in the older person	148
6.2	Observable indicators of the potential presence of pain in cognitively impaired older people	150
6.3	Pain assessment tools to aid pain management for the nonverbal older adult	153
6.4	Examples of pain assessment tools and age range of infants tested	159
6.5	CRIES pain assessment tool	160
6.6	CHEOPS assessment categories	160
6.7	General guidelines for the management of pain in neonates, infants and children	162
7.1	A guide to the management of sickle-cell disease pain	183

Foreword

Pain is a common experience for many people. Approximately 1 in 7 people in the UK live with chronic pain (Chronic Pain Policy Coalition 2007) and 78% of visits to the A&E are due to pain (Wagner 2008). Persistent pain following common surgeries such as groin hernia repair, breast and thoracic surgery, leg amputation, and coronary artery bypass surgery is fairly common, occurring in 10–50% of patients (Nikolajsen et al. 2006). Pain has significant effects on the individual's quality of life, affecting the ability to work, social activities and common daily activities such as exercising, sleeping, walking and sexual relations.

As someone who is involved in the education of health professionals, I have been looking forward to the second edition of this book. In some areas, the field of pain management has undergone significant developments in the eight years since the first edition. Our expanding understanding of the complexities of pain physiology with the use of modern imaging techniques and our developing understanding of the psychological and emotional components of the pain experience have further emphasised the importance of a biopsychosocial model of pain. Recent research has highlighted the complexity of the way pain perception occurs and the areas of the brain that are involved. The importance of the emotional centres in the brain in modifying pain-related nervous system messages and in producing the pain experience increasingly highlights the role of emotion in the perception of pain. The complexity of the nervous system that is responsible for the experience of pain further highlights the need to treat pain on an individual basis and the importance of pain assessment.

In practice, these developments have been matched by the further development of services and techniques in acute and chronic pain. However, despite these developments, there is still evidence of unrelieved pain in acute settings and in those with long-term conditions, particularly vulnerable groups such as older people, children and those with learning difficulties. The reasons for this are complex but a clear finding of much research is an educational deficit among healthcare practitioners in relation to pain. This was recognised in the 'new pain manifesto' launched by the Chronic Pain Policy Coalition (2007), which highlighted the need for education to be an integral part of all professional training.

The updated version of this innovative book therefore comes at an important time. It aims not just to provide information about the assessment and management of pain, but to present it in an interactive and structured way that provides a useful education experience. This edition will challenge and stimulate the reader to take the knowledge provided and reflect on their own practice and, more importantly, to apply this learning to their own practice and thus improve pain assessment and management. The authors also provide useful practical resources for the reader, including assessment charts, algorithms and prescription labels.

There can be no greater reward for healthcare practitioners than to relieve the pain and suffering of those under their care, and this book will contribute to their ability to achieve this. The authors are two of the most respected practitioners and researchers in the field of pain and their approach to the integration of theory and practice is reflected in the structure of this text. Improved knowledge about pain will do little to improve patient experience in itself unless it is applied to practice. The approach taken here – to help the reader to relate the substantial body of information about pain assessment and management to their everyday practice – will help to overcome this.

Dr Nick Allcock

Chronic Pain Policy Coalition (2007) A new pain manifesto, http://www.paincoalition. org.uk/.

Nikolajsen L., Brandsborg B., Lucht U., Jensen T.S. and Kehlet H. (2006) Chronic pain following total hip arthroplasty: A nationwide questionnaire study. Acta Anaesthesioligica Scandinavica, **50**(4): 495–500.

Wagner J.M. (2008) Acute Pain in the Emergency Department: *Clinical Practice, Research, and Development,* http://medscape.com/viewarticle/576475.

Preface

Reflecting back on our Preface eight years ago, there have been changes and improvements in pain management but these have not been far-reaching enough. Research documenting the undertreatment of pain can be found with regularity in the healthcare literature of the past 40 years and rarely a week passes without a story of unnecessary pain and suffering. Improvements in pain management have reached certain groups, but overall the problem of inadequate pain management persists across all age groups, cultures, hospitals and the community. Nurses have been charged with being the guardians of the quality of care (DH 2008) and pain management must be central to such endeavours.

Inadequate knowledge is recognised to be the most frequent reason for poor pain management, and education is probably the most important tool available to counteract this. You may read this unflinchingly, perhaps with acceptance, yet it would be different were we to write: 'Inadequate knowledge was again blamed for the error made by the captain, resulting in the third transatlantic plane plunging into the Atlantic last week.' There would be a national outcry, people would stop flying and (we imagine) a mandatory training initiative would be launched for all pilots to undertake. Pain education is often neglected in the undergraduate curricula, not just for nurses but across all professional groups. Yet pain is one of the main reasons that people consult their GPs and unfortunately pain continues to be an experience that so often accompanies any interaction with the healthcare services.

Competition for space in busy curricula is vigorous and pain is frequently not given a high priority. These challenges can be targets for our educational initiatives, but a question remains: how can education change practice? We set out, a few years ago, to deliver some pain units to experienced nurses working across a range of clinical areas. In our teaching, we included activities that encouraged them to collect information from their own clinical area and reflect on these findings along with those from research studies. The impact of bringing those two dimensions together was tremendous. Suddenly, there was an energy, created by the tension between what was happening in practice and what *might* happen in practice – the possibility, a vision. Bridging the disordered world of practice endorsed our student-centred approach in tackling pain education and, as they say, 'we haven't looked back.'

We hope you will enjoy this book and feel that we share your struggles and frustrations; more importantly, however, we hope it gives you the confidence to use the knowledge you have gleaned to provide the best possible care for those who suffer in pain.

EILEEN M. MANN
ELOISE C.J. CARR

DH (Department of Health) (2008) *Framing the Nursing and Midwifery Contribution: Driving up the Quality*. London, TSO.

Acknowledgements

Inspiration to take ideas and transform them into a book is not easy and many people have been influential on our journey. Close to home at Bournemouth University, the Clinical Leaders in Pain Scholarship group has provided enthusiasm and informed discussion which has helped enormously to develop the book; Jan Barrett, Ruth Day, Mandy Layzell, Rachael Weddell and Mary Pay.

Further afield, the British Pain Society's Special Interest Group in Pain Education has provided a stimulating national network, which has brought us into contact with others who are committed to improving pain management through education.

Importantly, our own students have shared our desire to improve pain management and enthusiastically used our novel approaches to learning; we are grateful to them for describing to us their experience.

Lynda Thompson at Palgrave Macmillan has kept us on track and been immensely supportive and Maggie Lythgoe our copy editor has been meticulous and great fun. With any endeavour of this sort, it is always our families to whom we owe so much. It is with genuine gratitude that we thank Peter and Tim for their selfless support, understanding and patience with our technical bafflement on the computer.

Every effort has been made to trace all the copyright holders but if any have been inadvertently overlooked the publishers will be pleased to make the necessary arrangements at the first opportunity.

Introduction

How this book is organised

This textbook has been structured around seven chapters, starting with the multidimensional nature of pain. It is important to work through Chapter 1 first as it forms the basis of the learning that follows. Before any strategies can be implemented to reduce pain, it is imperative that pain is carefully assessed as this forms the baseline for evaluation. Assessment is the linchpin of effective pain management, and we urge you to work through Chapter 2 next. We hope Chapter 3 on the barriers to effective pain management will inspire you to challenge traditional practice and make you want to implement change. You may then choose either acute (Chapter 4) or chronic pain (Chapter 5), whichever is most appropriate to your own learning and interest. Finally, Chapters 6 and 7 take a pragmatic view of how to manage pain with people who are vulnerable and those whose pain is challenging. With the exception of children and the older person, many of these groups do not receive regular mention in pain textbooks.

We have tried to provide realistic approaches and further reading to help you. Particularly where appropriate, we have tried to include electronic versions of text and guidelines that are accessible via the internet from sites such as:

- British Pain Society www.britishpainsociety.org
- Bandolier www.jr2.ox.ac.uk/bandolier/ with links to the Pain Site
- Cochrane Collaboration http://www.cochrane.org/
- International Association for the Study of Pain (IASP) www.iasp-pain.org/index.html
- National Guideline Clearinghouse www.guideline.gov

There is also a wealth of additional internet resources to help you to access online education in the form of lectures, journal articles and conference papers. We have suggested learning materials from useful sites, such as Medscape – www.medscape.com/home – that enable you to register your details and then access what is currently available. Medscape was developed in the USA to provide healthcare professionals with timely, comprehensive and relevant clinical information. This site will email you regularly with new topics, journal articles and also audio recordings, transcripts and slide presentations from well-known speakers. It will require you to set up a log-on name and password. Some of the other sites will also enable you to register for email advice when new material is published or available. This helps you to tailor your search for material and support to your personal needs and obtain them as soon as they are published electronically.

The PeerView Institute – http://www.peerview-institute.org/ntk/ntk.nsf/html/index.html – runs a Need to Know (NTK) Watch service, a free daily email newsletter developed in collaboration with more than 290,000 physicians. It contains the latest medical literature from over 2,000 peer-reviewed journals. A customisable monitored therapies tracker and the NTK Scored Science gives you the most important clinical content, as determined by peers. Registering could not be easier.

How to use this book

We suggest that you buy an A4 ring-binder, seven section dividers (one for each chapter) and a thick pad of A4 paper. As you work through each chapter, you can make notes and file them; it is also useful to have somewhere to put any references you follow up.

Each chapter begins with several learning outcomes. These are the goals of learning and you should, by the end of each chapter, be able to achieve them. We include some indicative reading to give you some background and understanding before you start the chapter.

Scattered through each chapter are a number of different features, as outlined below:

- *Activities:* Within the text are activities for you to complete, based on what you have just been reading. These are central to your learning and we strongly urge you to take some time to complete them. They will give you a much greater insight and understanding of the topic being discussed.
- *Time out:* These sections are designed to provide some 'thinking' time and a bit of space to jot down reflections on personal experience. They can be undertaken on your own, or better still with a colleague. We can learn much from the experience of others, and working together may help to open up discussion.
- *Case histories:* These are illustrations, usually from our own practice, that relate the experience of a person/family and their pain. There are usually some questions for you to reflect on at the end.
- *Coffee break:* It is important for you to have a break, so we have taken the liberty of providing you with an excuse.

Where possible, we have also included diagrams to simplify the text. Factual information may be listed in tables for clarity and quick reference.

At the end of each chapter is a further reading list, the references cited in each chapter appearing at the end of the book. It has not been our intention that you read everything but that you 'cherry pick' any items that will inform your own interests. We have tried to direct you to chapters, articles and internet sites that are both informative and well written.

How can I assess my own learning?

This is not a standard question, but we feel that it is helpful to gain some feedback on the work you have completed. At the end of each chapter are 10 multiple choice questions. Try to complete them before referring to the answers provided as they are a quick and simple way of assessing your understanding. If you are a registered nurse, remember that this work can contribute to your portfolio and will be useful evidence that you are fulfilling the requirements of PREP and keeping clinically up to date. We hope, too, that your study will be an enjoyable experience.

CHAPTER 1

The Multidimensional Nature of Pain

Learning outcomes

On completion of this chapter, the student will be able to:

■ Explore contemporary theories of pain

■ Relate the influence of gating mechanisms to the perception of pain

■ Describe the neurotransmission of pain, identifying the mode of action of two common analgesics

■ Critically discuss the physical, psychological and social influences affecting a person's experience of pain

---

Indicative reading

Galea M. (2002) Neuroanatomy of the nociceptive system, in Strong J., Unruh A., Wright A. and Baxter G. (eds) *Pain: A Textbook for Therapists,* Chapter 2. Edinburgh, Churchill Livingstone.

Godfrey H. (2005) Understanding pain, part 1: Physiology of pain. *British Journal of Nursing*, 14: 846–52.

Gudin J. (2004) Expanding our understanding of central sensitisation. Medscape Neurology & Neurosurgery, www.medscape.com/viewarticle/481798.

Eide P. (2000) Wind-up and the NMDA receptor complex from a clinical perspective. *European Journal of Pain*, 4: 5–15.

Mann E. and Carr E. (2006) *Pain Management (Essential Clinical Skills for Nurses).* Oxford, Blackwell Publishing.

McQuay H., *Pain and its control.* The Oxford Pain Site at Bandolier, www.jr2.ox.ac.uk/bandolier/booth/painpag/wisdom/C1html.

Okuse K. (2007) Pain signalling pathways: from cytokines to ion channels. *International Journal of Biochemistry and Cell Biology*, 39: 490–6.

The Wellcome Trust Pain website, Sensing damage, www.wellcome.ac.uk/en/pain/microsite/science.html.

Wright A. (2002) Neurophysiology of pain and pain modulation, in Strong J., Unruh A., Wright A. and Baxter G. (eds) *Pain: A Textbook for Therapists,* Chapter 3. Edinburgh, Churchill Livingstone.

Background

Pain is unlike any other sensation. It is not a single measurable response like blood pressure or pulse; for the person in pain, it is a total experience that cannot be objectively measured. The experience of pain does not depend only on the strength of the stimulus that has caused the painful sensation: an individual's pain perception also depends on how the brain is prepared to deal with the messages it is receiving.

These mechanisms can be subject to huge variation, not only from person to person, but also on a situational basis. They can depend on factors such as:

- a person's mood – are they unhappy, fearful or anxious?
- their memory of previous painful experiences
- how previous pain was dealt with and controlled
- the cause of the pain and what that might signify to the sufferer
- their cultural background and how they were brought up to view pain
- the time of day and what else is going on around them. Is their environment interesting or boring? Is pain being felt in the middle of the night?
- a person's genetic makeup may also be significant.

All these factors and more can alter how a painful stimulus is interpreted by the brain. The mechanisms of pain perception are extremely complex, and many attempts have been made to try and explain this complexity. This chapter explores the theoretical basis of pain perception and its relationship to *simple* neurophysiology. We then consider how contemporary theories relate to people actually experiencing pain and how these theories can enhance our understanding.

Why has pain been so misunderstood?

Ancient philosophers thought of pain as an emotion, an imbalance of body fluids or a visitation from an evil spirit. The heart was seen as the centre of the painful experience. These simplistic theories of pain perception were held until quite recently.

A principle theory was based on the writings of the seventeenth-century philosopher Descartes. He described pain as being like a spark from a fire that stimulated threads in the skin to operate 'bells' in the brain – a straight channel from the skin to the brain. Even though the complex layout of nerve pathways had been recognised by anatomists for a long time, this simplistic idea of a message travelling directly from the site of pain to the brain was only seriously challenged around 40 years ago.

Science has been slow to tackle the problems of pain perception, but science alone is not to blame for this situation: many factors, such as social attitudes to pain and cultural beliefs, have resulted in pain being poorly understood and ineffectively controlled. For centuries, these attitudes and beliefs encouraged people to accept that pain was in some way beneficial, spiritually enhancing, character building or an unavoidable part of disease or injury. Now that we recognise that analgesia and positive pain control strategies – rather than pain – offer tangible benefits, we are beginning to see positive outcomes from effective pain control (Kehlet and Holte 2001). Perhaps more to the point, improved data collection and a growing awareness of the mechanisms of pain suggest there are linkages between poor acute pain control and a risk of serious morbidity (Royal College of Surgeons and the College of Anaesthetists 1990) and even chronic pain (Bandolier 2002).

Because pain perception varies widely between and also within individuals, it is possible to understand that Descartes' simple 'hard-wired' system could not possibly be correct; the mechanisms of pain perception are far more complex than this. It was only in 1965 that Professors Melzack and Wall published their first paper on a new theory of pain – gate control theory – that was to revolutionise the basic concepts of pain physiology.

 Time out

Think about a pain experience you have had. What was the cause of the pain? Consider the quality, intensity and location of this pain. How did it make you feel?

Everyone has at some time experienced pain. A major national survey of hospital patients undertaken in 1994 revealed that 3,163 (61%) of patients suffered pain, of whom 1,042 (33%) were in pain all or most of the time (Bruster et al. 1994). Although this is now somewhat dated, more recent data continue to suggest that the management of pain in hospitals is far from optimum. A survey conducted in 18 English hospitals in 2002 revealed that 24 hours after surgery, 22% of patients experienced moderate to severe pain even at rest, while 39% reported moderate pain on movement seven days following surgery (Taverner, 2003).

In the area of day case surgery, where pain is envisaged and should be relatively easy to control, a review by Wu et al. (2002) concluded that, on average, 45% of day case patients experience pain after surgery. A further study by McHugh and Thoms (2002) suggested that severe pain was a problem for 21% of patients two days post-operatively and this delayed recovery. Not only does pain delay recovery but a more serious consequence is that a percentage of patients will develop chronic pain following surgery. Patients are particularly at risk after procedures such as thoracotomy and hernia repair, with the data suggesting a strong link between poor pain control and this risk of pain chronicity (Callesen et al. 1999; Bandolier 2002; Page 2005).

Pain in the community is more difficult to estimate, but some work has been carried out. In a large study undertaken in Scotland in 1999, slightly over 50% of people reported some form of chronic pain (Elliot et al. 1999). More recent research from Denmark suggests an overall chronic pain prevalence of 19%, but this research also highlighted the negative consequences to the sufferer, their families and society in general. The odds of quitting one's job because of ill health were seven times higher among people experiencing chronic pain. This group also reported poor self-rated health and had twice as many contacts with various health professionals compared to the control group (Eriksen et al. 2003).

For cancer pain, the research paints a particularly disturbing picture. The World Health Organization (WHO), for example, conservatively estimated in the early 1990s that pain associated with cancer was experienced by at least 4 million people, with many not receiving satisfactory treatment (Foley 1993). In 2007, the situation remains problematic, a systematic review of the literature concluding that a substantial proportion of cancer patients suffer from moderate-to-severe pain and do not receive adequate pain treatment (van den Beuken-van Everdingen et al. 2007). Among the elderly population, the figures can be equally bleak, one study revealing that 45–80% of residents in a long-term care facility in the USA suffered from 'significant' pain (Loeb 1999).

In the previous time out, were you able to identify what 'type' of pain experience you were recalling? The first obvious type is either 'acute' or 'chronic'. **Acute pain** has a sudden onset and foreseeable end, and is associated with trauma or acute disease such as appendicitis or **cholecystitis**. Conversely, **chronic pain** is usually described as having lasted for more than three months, although this is seen by many as being far too simplistic (Waddell 1997). What is not in dispute is the fact that pain affects many aspects of a person's life, for example mood, sleep, mobility and relationships with other people.

We will be studying acute and chronic pain in later sections of this chapter, although at this stage it might be useful to stress that chronic pain is not just an acute pain that hasn't got better. It might include some of the inflammatory mechanisms associated with acute pain, but may also be associated with nerve damage, nerve dysfunction or alterations and 'remapping' within the central nervous system itself. Chronic pain also has the potential for massive psychological fallout as patients face up to the reality that they may have to live with pain for the rest of their lives.

Chronic pain may be associated with a degenerative ongoing condition such as **osteoarthritis**, or, quite frustratingly, it may be associated with no obvious organic pathology such as migraine headache or irritable bowel syndrome (IBS). In some cases, chronic pain can be completely unexplained by any medically identifiable condition, which isn't to say that it is not felt as a very real pain, but the reason for this pain, or the pain generator, can remain elusive and therefore difficult to treat.

Although pain is usually described as acute or chronic, there are many other descriptors of pain including **nociceptive**, **neuropathic**, **tractable/intractable**, **acute on chronic**, **persistent/persistent intermittent**, **referred**, **somatic**, **visceral** and **phantom**. (See the Glossary for definitions of these terms as it is important to understand what type of pain you are encountering before embarking on the search for its cause and potential treatment.)

The management of pain will continue to dominate our lives, for several reasons. With ageing populations, the incidences of degenerative diseases such as osteoarthritis will steadily increase. Also, many people now survive diseases that would once have killed them, and often live with conditions such as cancer, **multiple sclerosis (MS)**, **cystic fibrosis (CF)** and **systemic lupus erythematosus (SLE)**.

Newer diseases, such as **human immunodeficiency virus (HIV)** and **acquired immune deficiency syndrome (AIDS)**, can also lead patients to present with considerable pain problems.

So how can current theories of pain help us to understand people's pain experience? Gate control theory brought together all the anatomical, physiological, biochemical and psychological data available in the 1960s. Despite some modification, the theory has stood the test of time and will be covered in greater depth later on. Initially, we will explore the basic neurophysiology of pain and consider how gate control theory has been fundamental in helping us to understand the impact of acute pain. We then briefly explore a more recent theory termed 'neuromatrix', which offers a hypothesis about the development and lived experience of more enduring pain. First, it is helpful to define what we actually mean by pain.

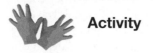 **Activity**

Think about what the term 'pain' means to you. Make some notes on how you would describe pain. Try to write only about what pain is, avoid writing about how it affects you.

Many people have attempted to define pain, and it is helpful to have a definition. McCaffery and Beebe (1994, p. 15) defined pain as:

whatever the experiencing person says it is and existing whenever he says it does.

The International Association for the Study of Pain (IASP 1986, p. 5216) offers another definition:

an unpleasant sensory and emotional experience associated with actual or potential tissue damage, or described in terms of such damage.

What we do know about pain, however, is that it is a subjective experience shaped by our previous pain history and is completely individual to the sufferer.

 Time out

Think about these two definitions. How helpful are they to your practice? Ask a couple of colleagues for their views.

McCaffery and Beebe's definition is making a statement about the uniqueness of an individual's pain and always believing the patient. Adopting the stance that you always believe the patient is fundamental for effective pain management. However, it does little to tell us about the experience of pain, which is clearer in the second definition. The latter also reflects a multidimensional understanding of pain that fits better with current pain theory.

An introduction to neurophysiology

Trauma, surgery and inflammatory disease cause a reaction at the site of tissue disruption or damage, and a physiological response throughout the body. The damage to tissue results in the release or production of a mass of chemicals, which react with each other and on nerve endings. This process has been colourfully described as a 'biological nuclear reaction' and the chemicals that result as an 'inflammatory chemical soup'. When these chemicals have stimulated the nerve endings, signals travel to the **dorsal horn of the spinal cord** and then up to the cortex of the brain, where the perception of pain takes place. Readers who wish to explore this in greater depth can refer to the indicative reading section.

Pain fibres or nociceptors

Looking at the actual nerves themselves, nerves have been classified according to what kind of message they convey, their size and the conduction rates of their fibres. There are three types of nerve fibre that are of particular interest to us. Two transmit pain sensation – the A delta and C fibres – while the A beta nerves transmit other sensations that are not normally painful, for example warmth and touch.

A delta fibres

When stimulated, these nerves transmit quickly and result in the instant reflex response that will cause the rapid withdrawal of tissue from a source of damage. Imagine putting your hand on the hot plate of a cooker. You remove it so rapidly that you are not consciously aware of your movement. The pain is instant, sharp and localised. This type of sensation carried by the A delta fibres is called 'first' or 'fast' pain.

The fibres travel to the dorsal horn of the spinal cord, which is divided into layers of cells termed **laminae**. These laminae have been numbered according to their location. After terminating mainly in lamina 1, the nerves give off long fibres that cross to the other side of the cord and then travel to the **thalamus** and **somatosensory** areas of the **cortex of the brain** (Figure 1.1). Because the A delta fibres end in the 'thinking part' of the cortex, we can fairly accurately localise the pain.

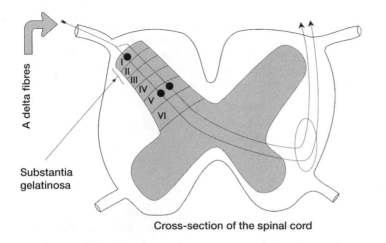

Cross-section of the spinal cord

Figure 1.1 The synaptic activity of A delta fibres in the spinal cord

It is these fibres that are also responsible for pinprick sensation. Interestingly, they do not have opioid receptors on their surface so do not respond to morphine-type analgesia. Nurses seem to have known this for a long time as patients who have been made comfortable with morphine will still experience the unpleasant sensation of being pricked with a needle. Patients will jump with pain, as they have not been rendered insensible to this sensation just because a previous pain has now been brought under control. This 'first pain' is still intact as a protective mechanism to ensure that tissue is not exposed to further potential damage. It is only by administering a **nerve block** or rendering a patient deeply anaesthetised that this protective reflex can be blocked.

Understanding this aspect of pain transmission is important as many patients are left in pain for hours under the mistaken impression that analgesics will 'mask' all pain and make diagnosis more difficult. This is not correct as the tenderness and pain sensation carried by the A delta fibres will not be affected by opioids. When pain has been well controlled but suddenly becomes uncontrolled despite regular, previously effective medication, alarm bells should ring. It could be heralding something serious to cause this change, and the patient's condition should be investigated further.

Case history

John Casey is a 28-year-old college student who was admitted to A&E with a 24-hour history of nausea and vomiting and right-sided abdominal pain. His general practitioner had given him 10mg morphine intramuscularly at 3 p.m., and he has received no further analgesia. It is now 6 p.m. and you have just taken over John's care. You have found him very distressed and he has rated his pain intensity as 9/10 on a 0–10 scale, 0 being equal to no pain and 10 representing the worst pain ever experienced (see Chapter 2). You notice that his prescription chart has no strong analgesia prescribed, and the house officer is reluctant to prescribe any until John has been examined by the senior registrar. The house office writes a prescription for a NSAID such as ibuprofen, which you feel will not provide adequate or rapid analgesia as John was taking NSAIDs with little effect prior to calling his GP. You are told that John will probably be going to theatre within the next few hours. How do you think you might overcome this problem?

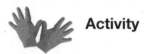 **Activity**

Talk to colleagues and get them to relate some of their experiences of either their own pain management, or an incident where they felt pain management could have been improved, particularly within a healthcare setting. Can you make a list of any other situations in which patients might wait in pain unnecessarily? Try making two lists, one covering misconceptions and one covering practice issues (refer to Chapter 3 if you need some help).

An accurate assessment of pain can help with the diagnosis, but denying effective analgesia until a diagnosis has been made can result in unnecessary suffering. An inflamed appendix is painful, and although morphine will make the patient more comfortable, if you prod the inflamed area, the patient will still complain. It might be helpful to ask for a trial of intravenous strong analgesia such as morphine **titrated** to response for patients like John. This would help medical staff to feel more confident that analgesia, when used appropriately, does not mask the diagnosis yet offers safe and acceptable pain relief for the patient.

C fibres

These fibres conduct impulses more slowly than A delta fibres and are associated with 'second pain', the dull, burning, aching, throbbing pain that is felt over a wider area. These slower pain fibres terminate in laminae 1 and 2 (the **substantia gelatinosa**) of the spinal cord and have short connecting fibres to lamina 5 (Figure 1.2).

The C fibres then generally follow the same pathway as the A delta fibres but terminate over a wide area within the brain stem. No fibres project into the somatosensory cortex of the brain, and patients report the pain as being more generalised. The good news is that this C fibre pain can almost always be subdued by the use of **opioids**, which is why this group of analgesics can be so effective in treating acute pain. How opioids achieve this will be covered later in this chapter.

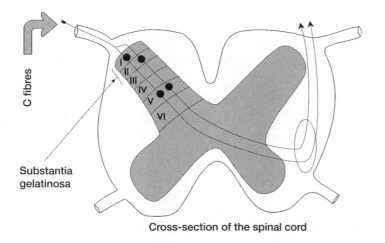

Cross-section of the spinal cord

Figure 1.2 The synaptic activity of C fibres in the spinal cord

Non-pain sensation

A beta fibres

Although not directly related to the transmission of painful stimuli, these fibres are worth mentioning here. Like pain fibres, there are many of them, and they are concentrated in the skin. They are the largest of the three fibres, do not cross over to the other side of the spinal cord and are the most rapidly conducting (Figure 1.3). These fibres are activated by touch and sensation that in a normal state would not be perceived as painful. Their significance will become clear when we study gate control theory in more detail.

Figure 1.4 illustrates how the nerve fibres described earlier transmit different sensations. All enter the dorsal horn of the spinal cord at the same point, the A delta and C fibres then crossing over to the other side before travelling up to the brain. The A beta fibres do not cross over but fast-track to the brain on the same side as they enter.

 Time out

Think again about pain relief other than that provided by the usual analgesics. Can you think of specific physical or psychological remedies that work well to relieve pain?

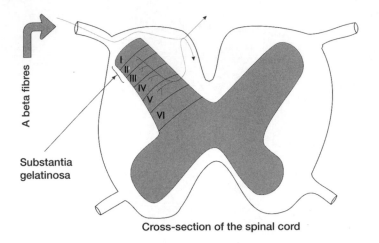

Figure 1.3 Activity of A beta fibres in the spinal cord

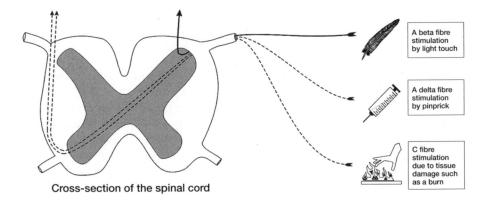

Figure 1.4 Touch, pinprick and burning sensations transmitted to the brain via the dorsal horn of the spinal cord

Gate control theory

Think about the following everyday scenario. We will then endeavour to explain this process using gate control theory and what is understood about the three nerve fibres that have just been described.

Case history

Olivia and Angela are playing at their classmate's fifth birthday party when Olivia falls heavily off the climbing frame. For a moment she is quite shocked and then realises she has hurt her leg. Olivia's mum is nearby and, hearing the cries, scoops her daughter off the ground and cuddles her. When she sees the bruising appearing on Olivia's leg, she gently rubs the affected area, still cuddling her. A few minutes later Olivia is back with her friend, playing happily.

Although there have been several theories to explain the nature of pain, the most influential has been gate control theory (Figure 1.5), originally proposed by Melzack and Wall in 1965 and continually updated by further research (Wall and Melzack 1994; McMahon and Kolzenburg 2005).

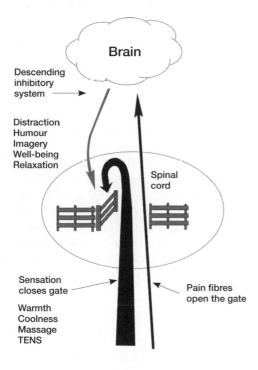

Figure 1.5 Gate control theory: how a gate may be opened or closed

Their theory explains the multidimensional nature of pain, reflecting the physiological, **cognitive** and emotional aspects of the pain experience, and offers explanations for phenomena that are complex in nature.

To recap, tissue damage results in a volley of nociceptive impulses that travel along small myelinated A delta nerve fibres and unmyelinated C fibres, which then synapse with cells in the substantia gelatinosa of the dorsal horn of the spinal cord. If inhibitory impulses are not initiated from either the periphery or the brain to close the 'gate', these impulses continue to ascend to the cortex, where the pain is perceived.

A major component of gate control theory refers to the mechanisms by which the peripheral and central nervous systems are able to modulate pain, either reducing or increasing the pain that is perceived. This modulation of pain takes place at two levels: at the level of the dorsal horn of the spinal cord where pain sensation may be altered by the stimulation of non-pain-transmitting nerve fibres from the periphery, or from cognitive or higher centres of the brain via fibres descending to the spinal 'gating' system. Pain perception can be altered by factors such as anxiety, excitement and anticipation that may open the 'gate' and therefore increase the perception of pain. Conversely, cognitive activities such as distraction, suggestion, relaxation, **biofeedback** and imagery help to close the 'gate' and prevent the sensory transmission of pain (Wall and Melzack 1999). The modulation that takes place at the dorsal horn level comes from the activation of the non-pain-transmitting A beta fibres. This can be achieved with stimulation such as a cold compress or rubbing the affected area.

To explain this more easily, think back to Olivia banging her shin, which is hurting. Her mother rubs the sore area vigorously but gently. This stimulates the fast-acting A beta fibres (the touch sensation fibres), which then feed into the dorsal horn of the spinal cord, where they synapse in the same area as the pain-transmitting fibres (the substantia gelatinosa). This area is a bit like a major traffic junction: if too many vehicles, in this case too many nerve impulses, arrive at the same time, some of the traffic gets clogged up. Only the swift traffic, in this case the sensation travelling via A beta fibres, taking the shortest possible route is likely to get through unhindered. Hence, when Olivia's mother rubs her daughter's injured shin, she creates a sensation of warmth and touch, effectively inhibiting the pain sensation from reaching the brain. Just as additional vehicles will hinder traffic at a roundabout, smaller faster vehicles can perhaps squeeze through. Distracting her with attention and a cuddle helps to allay Olivia's anxiety, acting on the cognitive features of the gate control mechanism further up the central nervous system, which are then stimulated to help to modulate the pain further and reduce its impact on Olivia.

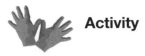 **Activity**

In the previous time out, you were asked whether you could think of specific physical or psychological remedies that work well to relieve pain. Now we have introduced this concept of a gating mechanism, can you think of any more examples of these interventions to reduce the pain experience? It may be helpful to make two lists, one headed 'pharmacological strategies' and one headed 'non-pharmacological strategies'. What particularly has worked for you?

Pain chemicals

Nerve cells have **receptors** on their surface, which react with or bind to a variety of chemicals found in the 'inflammatory soup' produced by trauma. Some of these chemicals – such as **substance P**, **bradykinin** and the **leukotrienes** – provoke the sensation of pain. Once this 'chemical cascade' has commenced, the inflamed tissue and its surrounding area becomes increasingly sensitised to pain by the production of **prostaglandins**, particularly prostaglandin E. This increase in pain is often termed **primary hyperalgesia**. These chemicals increase the pain transmission to higher centres, the painful area continues to become more sensitive and this sensitivity begins to spread to surrounding tissue, leading to **secondary hyperalgesia**. Other chemicals can actually reduce pain or remove pain sensation altogether. Confusingly, the action of these chemicals is often referred to as pain 'modulation', although modulation may, in fact, describe an increase as well as a decrease in pain.

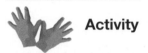 **Activity**

Look up non-steroidal anti-inflammatory drugs (NSAIDs) and make some notes on how they work or alternatively refer to the section in Chapter 4.

Case history

Mrs Jones, an elderly woman, lives alone in a small cottage on the edge of her son's farm. The district nurse has been visiting Mrs Jones for a few days to dress a wound on her leg. Yesterday she went in and Mrs Jones winced and cried out as she gently removed the bandage and was extremely distressed by the pain. The nurse was rather shocked as she had been very careful not to tug on the dressing and Mrs Jones's pain seemed out of proportion to the degree of tissue damage.

Reflect on the situation just described. What would you have done? Why had Mrs Jones become sensitive to having the dressings changed? What might help the pain in this situation?

Non-steroidal anti-inflammatory drugs (NSAIDs)

You will find that NSAIDs work by inhibiting an enzyme called **cyclo-oxygenase (COX)**, which is responsible for the production of prostaglandin. By inhibiting prostaglandin production, pain intensity is decreased. Unfortunately, one of the downsides of NSAIDs is their ability to block *all* cyclo-oxygenase enzymes. These include those enzymes needed for general housekeeping such as the production of the

mucosa that protects the stomach and small intestine, as well as chemicals that maintain renal function and platelet adhesiveness (Carr and Goudas 1999).

Opioids

One important group of receptors, which bind opioid-like chemicals produced in the
body, are known as the 'endogenous opioid receptors'. Clinicians administer chemicals that mimic endogenous opioids in order to reduce pain sensation. These chemicals are able to suppress conduction in the pain pathway and reduce the perception
of pain; this is the basis of opioid activity.

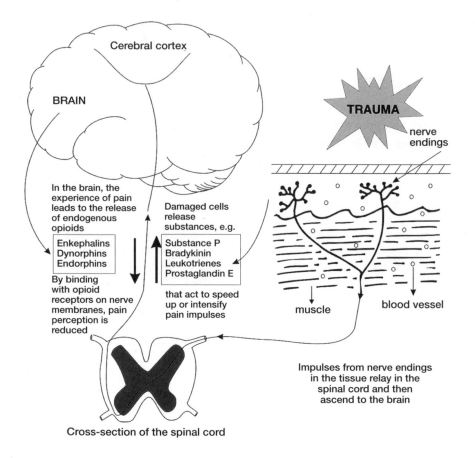

Figure 1.6 Response to the chemical cascade caused by tissue damage

Science has isolated chemicals produced as a result of trauma that can increase
pain, but the body also produces opioid-like substances and other **neurotransmitters**

that can alleviate pain. For thousands of years, man has been aware of a substance that occurs naturally in certain poppies, which can also reduce pain. The opium poppy, *Papaver somniferum,* produces opium from the sap of its seed head. In the early part of the last century, a young German chemist isolated the opioid morphine from the sap of the opium poppy. Morphine is the 'gold standard' of pain relief and the substance with which other analgesics are compared.

As shown in Figure 1.6, endogenous opioids are morphine-like substances produced by the body. Table 1.1 lists the endogenous opioids produced by the body in response to painful stimuli, alongside some of the commonly administered opioids that are either extracted from the opium poppy or manufactured as synthetic copies to produce a similar effect.

Table 1.1 Endogenous opioids and commonly administered opioids

Endogenous opioids	Commonly administered opioids	
Enkephalins	Morphine Codeine	extracted from the poppy
Dynorphins	Diamorphine Oxycodone	semi-synthetic compounds
Endorphins	Methadone Fentanyl	synthetic compounds

We now look briefly at how some of the endogenous opioids and commonly administered opioid drugs actually work.

Opioid receptors are principally found in the brain and spinal cord. Opioids (such as those mentioned above) bind to one of three different types of receptor, each receptor having a slightly different action:

1. the mu receptor
2. the kappa receptor
3. the delta receptor (mu, kappa and delta being, respectively, the 12th, 10th and 4th letters of the Greek alphabet).

So far, the majority of opioid drugs in use are strongly active at the mu receptor. Unfortunately, mu receptor activity produces not only analgesia, but also unwanted side effects (Table 1.2). A few opioid analgesics act principally on the kappa receptor, producing slightly different, but often no less problematic, side effects. Table 1.2 shows that delta receptor activity is the only one to produce analgesia alone. This receptor responds to the enkaphalins, but researchers have yet to find a drug that will do the same and result only in analgesia.

Knowing a little more about how opioids work within the body will help you to understand why they are most effective in the management of acute pain and can in some cases also be used for specific chronic conditions. In the above case study on Mrs Jones, her pain might be reduced by a short course of NSAIDS to dampen the inflammatory soup and may even require the use of a short-acting opioid to help reduce the pain of dressing changes.

Table 1.2 Activity of opioids at the three receptor sites

Receptor	Response when activated	Endogenous opioid	Analgesic drug with a strong affinity
Mu	Analgesia, respiratory depression, pinpoint pupils, sedation, euphoria, reduced gastric activity, constipation, urinary retention	Endorphins	Morphine
Kappa	Analgesia, dysphoria, hallucinations, paranoia	Dynorphins	Buprenorphine
Delta	Analgesia	Enkephalins	No drug currently available

Figure 1.7 illustrates how opioids lock onto the various receptors. When an opioid is firmly locked, it causes an active biological response and is termed an 'agonist'. Although opioids can produce severe unwanted side effects, administering a substance termed an 'antagonist' can immediately reverse their activity. An antagonist is a substance that can occupy the same receptor but has no biological activity, thus blocking the receptor against the biologically active agonist. For example, if a patient is experiencing respiratory depression as a result of an overdose of opioid and naloxone (an opioid antagonist) is administered, the unwanted side effect is reversed and the patient's respiratory rate will revert to normal very rapidly. Unfortunately, if too much naloxone is given, over and above that needed to restore normal respiratory effort, all analgesic effects are reversed also and the pain will inevitably return.

Nurses give out many drugs, for example digoxin, against which there are no antagonists, so why do we get so anxious about the unwanted side effects of opioids? The fear of respiratory depression and addiction is often given as a reason for healthcare professionals being reluctant to prescribe and administer opioids. Research, however, indicates that these fears are unfounded, as fewer than 1% of patients suffer these unwanted side effects (Friedman 1990), and every opportunity should be taken to dispel these myths. For a more in-depth text on opioids, the reader is referred to McQuay (1999).

The psychosocial impact of pain

So far, we have considered several important aspects of neurophysiology that we know contribute to the perception of pain. However, explaining why fast and slow pains are different, as well as the effect that other sensations and chemicals may have on pain perception, does not account for some of the other anomalies that are associated with pain. Gate control theory helps to explain some of these by emphasising

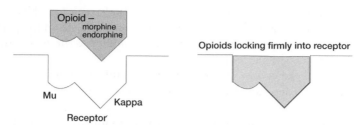

How opioids such as morphine lock onto receptors located on nerve membranes

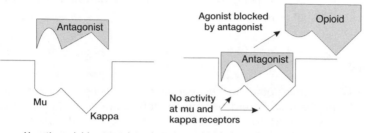

How the opioid antagonist naloxone can block the action of opioids

Figure 1.7 Receptor activity

the importance of pain modulation within the brain and at spinal cord level. It is ultimately the brain that dictates how much pain we feel from a potentially noxious stimulus, or whether, in fact, we feel any at all. This helps to explain:

- why some people appear to feel pain more than others after the same injury or following the same surgery
- why some people feel pain when there is no apparent injury
- why some people feel no pain when they have a serious injury, for example during active service in war zones
- why chronic pain can persist long after the original wound has healed or the initial cause of the pain has been removed.

Gate control theory provides an understanding for the use of some of our non-pharmacological interventions, such as relaxation therapy, transcutaneous nerve stimulation and other mind–body approaches (see Chapter 4), and has helped to explain many of the more baffling aspects of pain.

The great strength of gate control theory lies in the multidimensional framework it offers us and its adaptation or plasticity. **Plasticity** refers to how the peripheral and central nervous systems can be modified and show considerable adaptation to painful injury (Sluka and Rees 1997).

The three components of pain are:

- *Sensory-discriminative:* allows the injury, as well as the intensity of pain, to be identified in time and space.

- *Affective-motivational* (emotional): relates to how the body reacts to the pain in terms of its protective processes, for example in movement away from the painful stimulus. It is also concerned with how our emotions influence the motivational factors involved in our experience of pain.
- *Cognitive-evaluative:* explains how our response to painful stimulus is influenced by our cultural values, anxiety, attention and previous pain experience.

Gate control theory provides a multidimensional explanation for the individual experience of pain, involving all three components. This theory will feature throughout the book, so it is important to spend some time understanding it so that you can enjoy using this knowledge as you progress.

Case history

John Harding is an active father of two young children and regularly enjoys playing football with them on Saturday morning. John's father died from a heart attack when John was small and he worries that he too may die young. Last Saturday, as John was playing, he felt a slight discomfort in his chest and was suddenly overwhelmed with a sense of panic: 'what's this – a heart attack?' His pain got worse and he began to feel dizzy. He sat down and a friend called an ambulance. By now John was convinced the pain was a heart attack. Following an ECG and some blood tests, the news was good – not a heart attack. It must have been indigestion.

What factors served to increase the experience of pain for John. How could a slight chest pain escalate into something so serious as to make John convinced that he was having a heart attack?

 Time out

Think back to the pain experience you described at the start of this chapter. Can you identify any of the components of gate control theory described above?

You might find it useful to try the following activity. Our personal experience of, or preoccupation with, some of the points in this activity are believed to influence the descending modulatory or inhibitory pathways and how the brain responds to a painful stimulus.

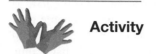 **Activity**

The following active thought processes within the brain influence the descending modulatory mechanism. Try to determine which component of gate control theory (for example cognitive-evaluative) these relate to.

Match the following thought processes to the components of gate control theory by writing in the box opposite:

- Memory of past events

- Boredom

- Emotional state

- Whether the pain is perceived to indicate serious or incurable disease

- Whether attention is being diverted by a more demanding thought process, as is the case with some individuals on active service in the forces or during a crucial rugby match

- How our culture and upbringing may influence our response to pain

- Whether you are being given a pleasant massage

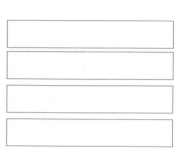

ANSWERS	Memory of past events:	predominantly cognitive-evaluative
Boredom:	predominantly cognitive-evaluative
Emotional state:	predominantly affective-motivational
Serious disease:	predominantly affective-motivational
Diverted attention:	predominantly cognitive-evaluative
Culture and upbringing:	predominantly cognitive-evaluative
Massage:	predominantly sensory-discriminatory

Most of the answers will actually involve a combination of the above, again illustrating pain's complexity. Can you see how some of these factors powerfully came into play with John's concerns about having a heart attack?

Pain often becomes more difficult to control when a person is frightened, for example when they have lost trust in those caring for them or have become over-whelmingly anxious. A combination of other factors may also amplify pain perception, such as feelings of not being in control or not knowing what is happening. Studies looking at the outcome of pain experienced during a time of acute stress, such as following a road traffic accident, are also revealing as they suggest a link between the stress response and persistent pain (Mclean et al. 2005). There are also studies that reinforce the need to prepare patients for pain particularly prior to surgery (Bandolier 1999). Some patients will try to use a range of coping mechanisms from wanting to know as much as possible to wanting to remain completely ignorant of what is happening to them. **Locus of control** can be an important concept to consider when preparing patients, as this may have an impact on the benefit of preoperative information-giving. Giving Mrs Jones (see earlier case study) the opportunity to remove her leg dressing would give her a greater sense of control and potentially reduce the pain.

We have discussed how pain can be regulated by both the peripheral and central nervous systems, sensitised by neurotransmitters that can be enhanced by negative thought processes which escalate pain. Conversely, we know that pain can be modulated downwards by endogenous chemicals, the use of analgesia, as well as strategies such as information-giving, touch, vibration, positive thinking, relaxation and other non-pharmacological coping strategies.

However, we also know that acute pain can become chronic for some individuals. Tissue damage can lead to a blurring of the boundaries between the sensations normally carried by A beta fibres and the pain sensations transmitted by C fibres, with the non-pain-transmitting A beta fibres acquiring the capacity to evoke pain, a condition termed **allodynia**. Pain and sensation fibres both become more easily stimulated, the receptive fields expand and there can be a loss of central inhibition via descending pathways. The consequences of these changes result in less stimuli proving painful, the pain lasting longer and spreading to uninjured tissue, a feature of secondary hyperalgesia.

Case history

Mrs Jones's pain continued to be difficult to manage but the nurses worked with her to find ways in which they could make the dressing changes more comfortable. Interestingly, it was the non-pharmacological interventions that seemed to make the difference. Mrs Jones enjoyed music so it was agreed she would choose a particular tape and this would be played during the visit. At the same time, a lavender aromatherapy candle was lit and the scent always provided a relaxing atmosphere. Each time the nurse changed the dressing, which Mrs Jones would remove first, she would ask Mrs Jones to relate a short story from her teaching days. Usually these distracted her sufficiently for the time to pass quickly.

Wind-up and hyperalgesia

Although there are many reasons why chronic pain may develop, researchers are currently becoming more interested in the consequences of unresolving secondary hyperalgesia and a condition that describes the dynamic plasticity of the nervous system referred to as **wind-up**. Wind-up and hyperalgesia may help to explain why the pain a person experiences sometimes seems worse than would be expected, becoming more intense and widespread than the damage causing it. This heightened response has recently attracted considerable scientific interest, as in some cases it may be implicated in the development of chronic pain syndrome (Eide 2000; Gudin 2004).

Consider wind-up as the result of nerve fibres transmitting painful impulses to the brain becoming 'trained' to deliver pain signals. Just like muscles get stronger with exercise, so the more nerves are stimulated, the more effective they become at transmitting signals. To make matters worse, the brain becomes more sensitive to the pain and shows expanded areas of response during sophisticated imaging. Although the terms 'wind-up' and 'secondary hyperalgesia' are not the same phenomena, they are sometimes used interchangeably and share common principals (see Glossary for further definitions).

Although it is not fully understood, it is believed that the activation of the **NMDA (N-methyl-D-aspartate acid) receptor** could be responsible for this unpleasant phenomenon. Many of the chronic pains encountered in pain clinics may be an end product of wind-up, pain occurring spontaneously and frequently, and persisting long after healing has taken place (McQuay and Dickenson 1990).

An understanding of wind-up may help to explain why pre-emptive analgesia, especially when pain is blocked by a local anaesthetic before it enters the spinal cord, may result in good postoperative analgesia for some patients. With the use of opioids and local anaesthetics, laboratory studies of individual nerve cultures indicate that the activity of nociceptors can be effectively suppressed. As any recovery nurse will tell you, however, once a painful sensation has reached the conscious brain, it takes a much higher dose of analgesia to suppress the stimulation.

Neuromatrix theory

Although acute pain can be explained well by gate control theory, gating mechanisms cannot explain some of the chronic pain we see in clinical practice, for instance the development of phantom limb pain or the complexity of pain experienced by paraplegics. The development of this sort of chronic or persistent pain appears to develop as a result of damage to the nervous system but amplified by psychological trauma and stress. The alterations that can take place within the nervous system associated with nerve damage or certain disease processes may be better explained by Professor Melzack's neuromatrix theory which he has continued to develop in the years since the death of his colleague Professor Wall.

The gate control theory emphasised the central nervous system's ability to filter, select and modulate inputs from the periphery. Melzack's (1999) neuromatrix theory emphasises the impact of brain function, proposing that the brain possesses a neural network, which he has termed 'the body-self neuromatrix'. This neuromatrix is predominantly genetically determined but integrates multiple inputs throughout our lives to produce the pattern that evokes an individual's pain – the **neurosignature**. Although the body-self neuromatrix is determined by sensory influences, it is also influenced by genetics and the network of nerves linking the somatosensory, **limbic** and thalamocortical components of the brain that integrate the sensory-discriminative, affective-motivational and cognitive-evaluative dimensions of pain experience.

The neurosignature output of the neuromatrix determines the particular qualities and other aspects of the pain experience and individual behaviour (Melzack 1999). It sounds complicated but is a fascinating theory and well worth reading more about as it is especially important for understanding phantom limb and other more complex chronic pain syndromes.

The multiple inputs of a pain experience that act on the neuromatrix contributing to the neurosignature include:

- sensory inputs (cutaneous, visceral and other somatic receptors)
- visual and other sensory inputs that influence the cognitive interpretation of the situation
- cognitive and emotional inputs from other areas of the brain
- intrinsic neural inhibitory modulation
- the activity of the body's stress regulation systems, including inflammatory, **endocrine**, **autonomic** and **immune response**
- the influence of an individual's opioid system.

The power of neuromatrix theory, although not universally accepted, is that it provides us with a framework in which a genetically determined template for the body-self is powerfully influenced by our cognitive function and our response to stress in addition to traditional sensory inputs. This theory may help to explain why some individuals develop chronic pain while others do not and why pain can develop in missing or damaged limbs.

Pain and suffering

There is an inevitability that when an individual experiences pain there will also be suffering. It seems the words are inextricably linked and it is perhaps the latter that makes those watching feel so helpless. Suffering pain can be seen as the inevitable sequelae to pain itself. Eric Cassell (2004) is one of the most cited authors on the nature of suffering and defines it as 'the state of severe distress associated with events that threaten the intactness of the person'. He later discusses a rich range of difficulties including the dilemma whereby a patient writhes on the X-ray table in pain, the X-ray shows an absence of disease, but the patient is clearly in pain (Cassell 2004). It is important to recognise suffering as integral to the experience of pain, wrapped up in the religious, spiritual and cultural traditions of the individual. So important is this concept that Patrick Wall wrote an elegant and poignant book when he was dying from cancer entitled *Pain: the Science of Suffering* (1999) – an inspirational book for both professionals and those with the misfortune to experience and suffer pain.

Conclusion

This chapter has explored some of the more complex aspects of pain, but hopefully you now have a clearer grasp of the subject that will help you to understand how pain is perceived and why it may change. These newer understandings suggest pain resides in a dynamic and plastic nervous system. Understanding the different mechanisms that contribute to a person's pain experience can help you to select interventions that exploit some of this knowledge and offer more effective pain relief. We hope the rest of this book will give you some tools to help to overcome some of the challenges of pain.

After a break, try the multiple choice test below in order to self-assess your understanding so far. For some of the questions, more than one answer will be correct, however, there will be one answer that is best supported by the evidence.

Suggested further reading

Carr D. and Goudas L. (1999) Acute pain. *Lancet*, **353**: 2051–8.
Kim H. and Dionne R. (2005) Genetics, Pain, and Analgesia. IASP Clinical Updates, September, XIII(3), www.iasp-pain.org/, click on Publications.
Lasch K. (2002) *Culture and Pain*. IASP Clinical Updates, December, X(5), www.iasp-pain.org/, click on Publications.
Melzack R. (1999) From the gate to the neuromatrix. *Pain*, Aug; Suppl 6: S121–6.
Melzack R. and Wall P. (1996) *The Challenge of Pain*, 2nd edn. Toronto, Penguin.
Melzack R. and Wall P. (2003) *Handbook of Pain Management: A Clinical Companion to Textbook of Pain*. Edinburgh, Churchill Livingstone.
Page G. (2005) Acute Pain and Immune Impairment. IASP Clinical Updates, March, XIII(1), www.iasp-pain.org/, click on Publications.
Vlaeyen J. and Crombez G. (2007) Fear and Pain. IASP Clinical Updates, August, XV(6), www.iasp-pain.org/, click on Publications.

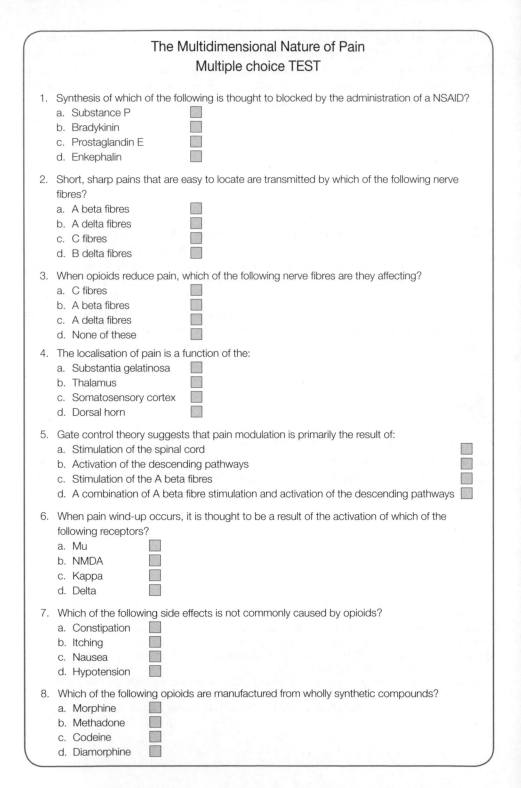

The Multidimensional Nature of Pain
Multiple choice TEST

1. Synthesis of which of the following is thought to blocked by the administration of a NSAID?
   a. Substance P ☐
   b. Bradykinin ☐
   c. Prostaglandin E ☐
   d. Enkephalin ☐

2. Short, sharp pains that are easy to locate are transmitted by which of the following nerve fibres?
   a. A beta fibres ☐
   b. A delta fibres ☐
   c. C fibres ☐
   d. B delta fibres ☐

3. When opioids reduce pain, which of the following nerve fibres are they affecting?
   a. C fibres ☐
   b. A beta fibres ☐
   c. A delta fibres ☐
   d. None of these ☐

4. The localisation of pain is a function of the:
   a. Substantia gelatinosa ☐
   b. Thalamus ☐
   c. Somatosensory cortex ☐
   d. Dorsal horn ☐

5. Gate control theory suggests that pain modulation is primarily the result of:
   a. Stimulation of the spinal cord ☐
   b. Activation of the descending pathways ☐
   c. Stimulation of the A beta fibres ☐
   d. A combination of A beta fibre stimulation and activation of the descending pathways ☐

6. When pain wind-up occurs, it is thought to be a result of the activation of which of the following receptors?
   a. Mu ☐
   b. NMDA ☐
   c. Kappa ☐
   d. Delta ☐

7. Which of the following side effects is not commonly caused by opioids?
   a. Constipation ☐
   b. Itching ☐
   c. Nausea ☐
   d. Hypotension ☐

8. Which of the following opioids are manufactured from wholly synthetic compounds?
   a. Morphine ☐
   b. Methadone ☐
   c. Codeine ☐
   d. Diamorphine ☐

9. Which of the following drugs will reverse the action of an opioid?
   a. Nalbuphine ☐
   b. Buprenorphine ☐
   c. Naloxone ☐
   d. Fentanyl ☐

10. Which of the following statements most closely describes neuromatrix theory?
    a. The emphasis is on the impact of brain function ☐
    b. Pain is genetically determined ☐
    c. Chronic pain develops as a result of the stress response ☐
    d. Chronic pain development is dependent on an individual's opioid system ☐

Answers

1. c. Prostaglandin E is the hormone-like substance that can be blocked by the administration of a NSAID.
2. b. A delta fibres transmit short, sharp, well-defined pain signals, C fibres generalised dull aching pain and A beta fibres sensations such as vibration and touch. B delta fibres do not exist.
3. a. C fibres; there are no opioid receptors located on the A delta or A beta nerve fibres.
4. c. The somatosensory cortex of the brain; the substantia gelatinosa is the area in the spinal cord where the modulation of pain occurs. The thalamus is a relay and coordinating station for sensory impulses, and the dorsal horn is the area where pain nerve fibres enter the spinal cord before they are relayed to the brain.
5. d. A combination of A beta fibre stimulation and activation of the descending pathways. All the others are also involved in pain modulation but d. gives the most comprehensive description of gate control theory.
6. b. The NMDA receptor; kappa, delta and mu are all types of opioid receptor.
7. d. Hypotension is rarely seen while all the others are common side effects of opioids.
8. b. Methadone; morphine and codeine are extracted from opium poppies and diamorphine is a semi-synthetic compound.
9. c. Naloxone; all the others are analgesics. Fentanyl is a pure agonist, buprenorphine and nalbuphine are opioids with agonist antagonist properties.
10. a. The emphasis is on brain function. Neuromatrix theory incorporates all the other factors but stresses the importance of the brain's unique 'neurosignature'. This is composed of patterns of nerve impulses generated by a widely distributed neural network – 'the body-self neuromatrix' in the brain.

CHAPTER 2

Assessing Pain

Learning outcomes

On completion of this chapter, the student will be able to:

■ Critically evaluate pain assessment tools and measures of pain currently in use for both chronic and acute pain

■ Discuss the importance of implementing pain assessment tools in clinical practice as a means of monitoring individual reports of pain and the acceptability, efficacy and safety of treatment

■ Review the influence of patient, professional and organisational factors on the effective implementation of pain assessment

Indicative reading

Bird J. (2003) Selection of pain measurement tools. *Nursing Standard*, **18**: 33–9.

Carr E. (1997) Assessing pain: a vital part of nursing care. *Nursing Times*, **93**(38) 46–8.

Fishman S. (2006) Breakthrough pain: strategies for effective assessment and the role of rapid-onset opioids in treatment, *Medscape*, http://www.medscape.com/viewprogram/6041.

Schofield P. (1995) Using assessment tools to help patients in pain. *Professional Nurse*, **10**(11): 703–6.

Schofield P. and Dunham M. (2003) Pain assessment: how far have we come in listening to our patients? *Professional Nurse*, **18**(5): 276–9.

Williamson A. and Hoggart B. (2005) Pain: a review of three commonly used pain rating scales. *Journal of Clinical Nursing*, **14**(7): 789–804.

Wood S. (2004) Factors influencing the selection of appropriate pain assessment tools. *Nursing Times*, **100**: 42–7.

Background

Evidence suggests that nurses' assessment of pain is limited as well as often being inaccurate (Carr 1997; Sjostrom et al. 2000). Nurses still tend to use their own judgement and prefer to rely on physiological signs and behaviours, which can be misleading (Drayer et al. 1999). Even in the postoperative setting where acute pain will respond well to analgesia and comfort measures, pain has been shown to go unnoticed or be inadequately managed (Sherwood et al. 2000; Dihle et al. 2006; Schoenwald and Clark 2006). While there is evidence that medical staff fail to prescribe effective analgesia, the problem is compounded by nurses administering medication, particularly opioids, at the lower end of the dosage range (Carr 1990). Further evidence suggests that they may also fail to negotiate a change of ineffective medication with medical staff (Valdix and Puntillo 1995; Cecilia 2000).

Interestingly, despite these many shortcomings, patients will often remain reluctant to complain about the levels of their postoperative pain (Schoenwald and Clarke 2006). There are many reasons for all these shortcomings and nurses are by no means entirely to blame. However, as nurses spend more time with patients in pain than any other health professional, they are in a powerful position to optimise pain control.

Formal pain assessment tools facilitate effective communication and assessment by reducing the chance of error or bias. An assessment tool that has been successfully implemented can provide compelling evidence of ineffective analgesia or unacceptable side effects that is hard to ignore. This chapter explores the nature of pain assessment by critically considering how pain can be assessed and the use of formal pain assessment tools.

Why assess pain?

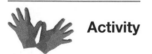 **Activity**

Take a minute to write down some of your thoughts on the question: Why assess pain?

If you are to manage pain effectively, it is imperative that you use an appropriate pain assessment tool rather than ask vague questions such as 'Anything for pain, Mr Smith?' as you peer over a drug trolley in an obvious hurry to finish the drug round. Conversely, a district nurse may elicit very little information if asking closed questions such as 'Have you any pain?' while visiting a patient who is sitting in their chair at home. These casual queries do not constitute a pain assessment and may even inhibit a truthful answer, as patients may feel that they cannot talk about their pain or it is of little importance. However, adequate assessment without effective management strategies will also result in poor quality care and frustration for professional, patient and carers. These are some of the advantages of using a formal pain assessment tool:

- provides patients with an opportunity to express their pain
- conveys genuine concern and interest about their pain
- helps to build a therapeutic relationship
- gives patients an active role in their pain management
- provides documented evidence of the efficacy or failure of any drugs or therapy provided
- reduces the potential risk of an overdose of medication
- enables the incidence of any side effects to be documented and their treatment evaluated
- reduces the chances of bias and error
- helps communication with other health professionals especially during staff changes.

Can you think of any other advantages of incorporating pain assessment into the general monitoring of patients?

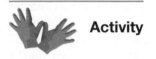 **Activity**

Approach a person you know who is experiencing pain or discomfort. Ask them if they are happy to discuss their pain. Find out what increases or reduces their pain. Ask them if they have ever had their pain formally assessed and did this improve their pain control. When you have finished, ask them how they felt about talking about their pain to you.

It is not possible to measure pain objectively in the clinical setting in the same way as we measure blood pressure; instead, we must mainly rely on subjective verbal methods. When communication with the patient is difficult, the observation of nonverbal communication and physiological responses is the only alternative. Assessment tools to help to assess these nonverbal indicators of pain have been developed, and many are currently in use to assess pain in infants, small children and the severely cognitively impaired. These tools are covered in greater depth in Chapter 6, but there is still a considerable way to go in their development so there is plenty of scope for creativity.

When to assess pain

Pain assessment should be integrated into the admission procedure for patients entering hospital particularly prior to surgery and should form part of an initial health assessment where patients have expressed pain as a concern or where it can be anticipated that a presenting condition may cause pain. For patients entering hospital with a painful condition, following trauma or for surgery that will inevitably result in pain, it is vital to obtain some baseline data. Patients might have pain that was not previously documented, the nurse can obtain some information about how pain has been managed in the past, previous experiences may be relevant, eliciting patients' expectations of pain management and maybe identifying personality features such as locus of control can be useful. A proactive approach has several advantages:

- Discussing pain assessment offers the opportunity to provide information to those patients who may find this beneficial (Shade 1992).
- Patient misconceptions can constitute a serious barrier to good pain management (Carr 1997). It is useful to be aware of these misconceptions before commencing therapy. Unfounded fears of addiction can seriously hamper even the best efforts to control pain.
- The nurse will be able to identify important issues that will improve pain assessment and management or provide a warning of issues such as high levels of anxiety or fear that may make effective pain control more of a challenge.
- Previous pain experiences can influence patients' expectations of how their pain will be managed; some may have particularly unpleasant memories.
- The suitability of a pain assessment tool can be checked before it is used. This is particularly important with children who might prefer to use a 'faces' scale rather than a verbal or numerical scale. Some people will have a problem conceptualising pain in a numerical or linear way so using a verbal description for pain intensity may suit them better.
- For nonverbal patients, a discussion with family or carers may help when selecting or modifying a pain assessment tool.
- Now is a good time to stress to the patient that pain is not considered to be an inevitable part of being a patient and that there are plenty of ways to control it.

How to assess pain

Verbal communication

Where possible, verbal assessment is the most accurate; this is the principal method unless a patient's age or condition makes it impossible. As stated earlier, assessment should commence as early as possible, for example preoperatively, as it can be valuable to establish the patient's expectation of pain relief. This is unfortunately often very low. People frequently come into hospital expecting pain from operations, tests or investigative procedures. Sadly, we usually give them what they expect, so on satisfaction surveys, patients are satisfied with their care. Even when patients have memories of considerable pain, they still report being satisfied with their pain relief as they got what they expected ... pain.

Communication is vital if the situation is going to improve, and it needs be a two-way process. The patient must be provided with suitable information regarding the various pain-relieving therapies that are available, and information must be obtained on patients' expectations of pain relief. It is also important to inform patients of the benefits of effective pain control, for example to allow them to mobilise or cough, and to prevent unwanted side effects. Too often, patients will resist taking analgesia and think that as long as they keep still and do not move, they will not experience pain. Unfortunately, it is this very immobility that can sometimes lead to life-threatening side effects such as **deep vein thrombosis (DVT)** and chest infection but many patients will be unaware of these risks.

In the community, particularly for patients with chronic pain, appropriate assessment should be integral to managing care but in practice pain assessment is rarely made explicit. This can lead to pharmacological and non-pharmacological strategies never being properly evaluated or an appropriate therapy being discontinued, as side effects were never addressed or patients' misconceptions left to hinder effective interventions. For patients undergoing painful procedures particularly in the community, a simple assessment tool can make a huge difference to patients' pain experiences. It can enable far more effective therapy to be administered to control this 'incident' pain, which is elicited by healthcare professionals for treatments such as wound dressings and ulcer debridement.

Visual displays of pain

With patients unable to communicate verbally, for whatever reason, the nurse will have to rely on visual and physical signs of pain. As unlikely as it may seem, even those patients able to speak may not wish to communicate that they are in pain. They might, for example, fear that a report of pain could lead to them spending more time in hospital, or they might be denying their pain for fear of what that pain might signify. In such cases, nonverbal displays of pain may be useful. Visual signs might include:

- *body language*: limited movement or keeping very still, guarding parts of the body, an abnormal posture, a change in gait when walking or a change in stature, rocking, picking and restlessness
- *facial expression*: increased or decreased eye contact, tears, grimacing, muscle tension, an alarmed look, squinting eyes and clenched teeth
- *vocalisation*: sighing, crying, moaning, spontaneous noises, a change in pitch, impaired speech, verbal abuse, disjointed verbalisation and calling out
- *distance*: becoming quiet, withdrawn and uncommunicative
- *emotion*: worried looking, angry, sad or a change in mood
- *other*: a lack of interest in food and the environment, or a disrupted sleep pattern.

Physical signs of pain

Changes in physiological signs can support the patient's report of pain but should not (except in the unconscious patient) be used as the only measure, as patients physiologically adapt to pain quite quickly. These changes include:

- *physiological*: relative changes in blood pressure (up or down), pulse and respiration rate, sweating, pallor and nausea
- *physical*: in chronic pain, changes in limb size as a result of muscle wasting, neurological abnormalities, changes in temperature and colour, mottling of the skin of an affected limb or muscle spasm.

Case history

Mr Hall is an older gentleman who has been admitted to your ward with widespread cancer metastases. He is quiet, withdrawn and unable to concentrate for long. Mr Hall frequently grimaces and moans. Because of the onset of severe nausea in the past 48 hours, he has been unable to take his regular oral analgesia – 100 mg slow-release morphine every 12 hours with 6-hourly paracetamol. What information do you need in order to plan your care effectively?

Possible solution: You will need to assess the pain quickly and with the least number of questions. Tell the patient that, in order to obtain effective analgesia, you will need to ask a few questions but that you will keep them brief.

- Get the patient to indicate the location of the pain.
- Ask how long the pain has been there.
- Ask the patient to rate the severity of his pain on a scale of 0–10 (0 = no pain and 10 = worst pain imaginable). Remember that not everyone will be able to give a numerical rating: they may be unable to concentrate, or they may not understand the concept. A simple verbal rating, although less sensitive, is then more appropriate, taking, for example, the form 'Is your pain now mild, moderate or severe?'
- Ask the patient what he normally takes for his pain and any strategies he finds helpful.

With this minimal information, you will have established the location, duration and severity of the pain, as well as the dose of medication that would normally provide relief. While his nausea is being brought under control, his opioid intake can be re-established rapidly via a non-oral route, that is, intravenously, subcutaneously or sublingually. Paracetamol is also available as an intravenous preparation and the NSAID ibuprofen can be given as a sublingual melt. When re-establishing analgesia, non-opioids given with opioids are useful for their opioid-sparing effects and as part of multimodal therapy, which will be covered in later chapters.

Even with the use of an appropriate tool, assessing patients' pain may not be as straightforward as it seems. About 40% of cognitively intact patients experience some difficulty in expressing their level of pain (De Rond el al. 1999). Patients and clinicians may not speak the same language or if they do, patients' reports of pain are typically reinterpreted by clinicians in light of other factors such as demographics or the emotional, cognitive and medical characteristics of both the patient and clinician. There can be miscommunication because of cultural differences particularly where a tendency to underreport pain may be an issue (Keogh et al. 2005). Some individuals will just resign themselves to suffering (Weiner and Rudy 2002) or their pain may be so severe that they fail to communicate at all and become completely withdrawn.

Nurse factors affecting the assessment of pain

There is a need for nurses to be aware of how their own values and perceptions may influence the evaluation of another person's response to pain. If healthcare professionals hold misconceptions or anxieties regarding pain management, these must be addressed through education. Nurses can be strongly influenced by patients' behaviour, with research continuing to highlight discrepancies between patients' and nurses' rating of pain (Carr 1997; Schafheutle et al. 2001; Gunningberg and Idvall 2007). It has been suggested that patients draw on their personal experiences of actually feeling pain, while nurses may relate to pain by unconsciously drawing on their clinical experience of the multitude of patients they have cared for over the years (Sloman et al. 2004).

Other issues identified include poor pain education for all healthcare professionals, heavy workload, lack of staff, constant interruptions and having to address the competing demands of nurses, doctors and patients. Other subtle barriers to implementing pain assessment have also been identified such as a belief that patients exaggerate the intensity of their pain, and a lack of agreement between doctors and nurses in estimating a patient's pain. Also nurses may resist regular assessment of pain if they feel that a patient has not been prescribed effective medication and they lack the skills to negotiate an improvement of this. In terms of heavy workload, it could be argued that if pain control was managed pre-emptively following regular and routine assessment, more time could be freed up. More to the point, pain-free patients would be better able to mobilise and self-care (Kehlet and Dahl 2003).

Patient factors affecting the assessment of pain

As already mentioned, a person's age, gender, previous experience of pain and cultural background all influence pain perception. Nurses need to be aware of these influences and remain non-judgemental and unbiased in their assessment of another person's pain. It is important to be aware that pain behaviours may not always indicate the 'severity' of pain that a person is feeling. People experiencing pain may try to minimise their pain; they may not want to worry their family, they may be embarrassed, they may feel that it is better to bear the pain or worry that it may stop them going home from hospital, or they may harbour many other misconceptions about pain and its management. New research into patient experiences following day case surgery suggest that patients themselves may unintentionally sabotage efforts to improve pain control (Older et al. 2007); this will be covered in more detail in Chapter 3.

Age

The older person

Many older people 'hide' their pain, especially if it is chronic. At home, they may have developed good strategies to help them through the day, such as taking short walks or watching their favourite TV programme. Sadly, when they are admitted to hospital, these disappear and patients are left vulnerable and often unable to cope. The 'obvious' pain behaviours such as grimacing and frowning are often absent if pain has become chronic. In addition, sufferers may feel that it is not 'acceptable' to express their pain or that it is a sign of weakness. Nurses need a good knowledge of the expression of pain in this population if they are to recognise and manage it successfully.

Case history

Mrs Joan Morris is suffering from dementia and has been admitted to a rehabilitation ward for respite care while her daughter takes a few days' holiday. Mrs Morris initially settled well, but after a few days you notice that she is reluctant to sit in her chair and is constantly fidgeting and trying to get comfortable. When you ask her whether she has any pain, she nods but is unable to respond verbally. You noticed earlier that it took a couple of nurses to help her out of bed this morning, and her right hip seemed particularly stiff. Make notes on how you might assess Mrs Morris's pain.

Possible solution:

- In an ideal situation, a preassessment with Joan's daughter might have enabled you to list any behaviour that she felt might indicate pain.
- Make a brief list of the behaviours you observe when Joan is being moved or appears to be uncomfortable.
- Observe her facial expression and body movements.
- The fact that Joan nods in response to your question about pain means that it may be quite possible for you to obtain a regular self-report of pain using a simple pain assessment tool. If everything is explained carefully, it is often surprising how effectively patients, even those with severe cognitive impairment, can communicate pain, if they are given the chance.
- Try to identify any new pathology, worsening of known pathology or procedures that appear to cause pain.
- Start a trial of analgesia and observe Joan's response. Does she appear more comfortable and relaxed, or is she still displaying discomfort, which could also be

related to her sudden change of scenery and the anxiety that this might be causing.

- Read Chapter 7 of this book for some more information on pain assessment tools for the cognitively impaired.

Small children and neonates

Very small children have had their pain even more poorly managed than adults. Nagy (1998) studied the effect this had on the psychological state of nurses looking after neonates. The study revealed that a primary source of stress among these nurses was the lack of valid assessment tools. Thankfully, we are beginning to make some progress in this field and the assessment of pain in neonates and children is covered in more detail in Chapter 6.

Gender

Another factor extensively discussed in the literature is gender and its impact on pain experience. There is now some agreement among investigators that certain biological as well as psychosocial factors explain gender-related differences to pain and its treatment (Wiesenfeld-Hallin 2005). Gender is therefore an important variable, which should be taken into account when assessing pain (Vallerand and Polomano 2000) and may even lead to the development of gender-specific drug therapies in the future.

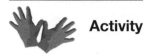 **Activity**

Ask a few friends or patients who they think feels pain more (men or women). Make a note of their responses. How could this influence the management of pain in practice? See whether you can find any literature on the subject. The use of vignettes in research would seem to indicate that many of us hold preconceived ideas.

Women who have given birth, and experienced intense pain, may be better able to cope with pain when they next experience it, especially if they felt in control at the time. It might also be argued that it is more acceptable for women than men to express their pain in an Anglo-Saxon-based culture. This might mean in practice that women 'appear' to suffer more pain than men if we are judging a person's pain by their behaviour.

Pain assessment tools

To capture formally information on patient's pain, a pain assessment tool is vital. The pain assessment tool should be valid, that is, there should be evidence that the tool is useful for the purpose intended, reliable and easily understood by the patient. For acute pain, which may change frequently, the assessment tool also needs to be quick and easy to use. We consider a range of different types of tool, including rating scales and questionnaires. Pain assessment particularly in the community setting or with vulnerable patients should also include the family or immediate carer. They will have a valuable insight into and understanding of the patient's pain experience, especially if there is cognitive impairment, hearing or visual difficulty.

The most reliable indicator of a person's pain and the distress it may be causing them is the patient's self-report. Self-report measurement scales include numerical or descriptive rating scales and visual analogue scales. A pain intensity score is a quick way of finding out the intensity of the pain for a given individual and evaluating the effectiveness of an intervention. Such scores are quick and simple to use, and most patients are able to understand them. The disadvantage of these scales is that they measure only intensity and give neither a description of the pain nor any additional information such as the degree of suffering the pain is causing. As a result they are often referred to as 'unidimensional' tools.

Visual analogue scale

This scale incorporates a 10 cm line, one end labelled 'No pain at all' and the other end labelled 'Worst pain imaginable' (Figure 2.1). Patients are asked to mark on the line the point corresponding to their pain. A pain score is then obtained by measuring, usually in millimetres, the distance between 'No pain at all' and the patient's mark. This can then give a precise figure and, when repeated later, can indicate small changes in pain intensity, which is particularly useful in research. This scale requires a patient to be able to concentrate. Some may have trouble understanding the concept, especially in the immediate postoperative period or following trauma when they may not feel particularly inclined to put marks on a line.

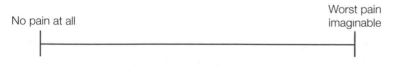

Figure 2.1 Visual analogue scale

Simple descriptive and numerical scales

These were the earliest of the pain assessment tools and simply use words, numbers or a combination of words and numbers to indicate the intensity of the pain or the effectiveness of any pain-relieving measures (Figure 2.2). They are easy to explain to patients and can be asked as a simple question.

Pain intensity

How bad is it?

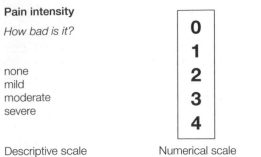

none
mild
moderate
severe

Descriptive scale   Numerical scale

Pain relief

How much relief has the treatment given?

none   (0)
slight   (1)
moderate   (2)
good   (3)
complete   (4)

Combination of both

Figure 2.2 Examples of pain scales

London Hospital pain observation chart

The London Hospital pain observation chart (Figure 2.3; Raiman 1986) was one of the earliest charts used in secondary care, developed with the aim of improving communication between the patient, the nurse and the doctor. The chart incorporates a body map, which can be particularly useful in pinpointing the source of pain (Latham, 1989). However, for regular everyday use, it may be too complicated. Introducing regular pain assessment into any area of healthcare can prove a real challenge and the simpler the tool, the more likely it will be used.

The London Pain Chart

Excruciating	5
Very severe	4
Severe	3
Moderate	2
Just noticeable	1
No pain at all	0
Patient sleeping	5

Left   Right   Right   Left

Date---------------- ✚ The London Hospital

Sheet number------ PAIN OBSERVATION CHART

TIME	PAIN RATING								MEASURES TO RELIEVE PAIN Specify where starred									Initials
	BY SITES								OVER-ALL	ANALGESIC GIVEN (name, dose, route, time)	Lifting	Turning	Massage	Distracting activities	Position change	Additional aids	Other	COMMENTS FROM PATIENTS AND / OR STAFF	
	A	B	C	D	E	F	G	H											

Figure 2.3 London Hospital pain observation chart
Source: Reproduced with kind permission of Mark Allen Publishing

Short-form McGill Pain Questionnaire

Melzack and Torgerson (1971) suggested that the words people chose to express their pain could form the basis of a multidimensional pain assessment tool. The McGill Pain Questionnaire (MPQ) is now one of the most utilised pain assessment tools in research studies and clinical practice across a range of painful conditions, particularly chronic pain. It has been translated into many languages around the world. Figure 2.4 displays the short-form version (SF-MPQ).

Patient's name		Date		
	None	Mild	Moderate	Severe
Throbbing	0)......	1)......	2)......	3)......
Shooting	0)......	1)......	2)......	3)......
Stabbing	0)......	1)......	2)......	3)......
Sharp	0)......	1)......	2)......	3)......
Cramping	0)......	1)......	2)......	3)......
Gnawing	0)......	1)......	2)......	3)......
Hot-burning	0)......	1)......	2)......	3)......
Aching	0)......	1)......	2)......	3)......
Heavy	0)......	1)......	2)......	3)......
Tender	0)......	1)......	2)......	3)......
Splitting	0)......	1)......	2)......	3)......
Tiring/exhausting	0)......	1)......	2)......	3)......
Sickening	0)......	1)......	2)......	3)......
Fearful	0)......	1)......	2)......	3)......
Punishing/cruel	0)......	1)......	2)......	3)......

No pain ◄————————————————► Worst possible pain

PPI

0 No pain	....
1 Mild	....
2 Discomforting	....
3 Distressing	....
4 Horrible	....
5 Excruciating	....

Descriptors 1–11 represent the sensory dimension of the pain experience and 12–15 the affective dimension. Each descriptor is ranked on an intensity scale of 0 = none, 1 = mild, 2 = moderate and 3 = severe. The present pain intensity (PPI) of the standard Long-form McGill Pain Questionnaire (LF-MPQ) and the visual analogue scale are also included to provide an overall intensity score.

Figure 2.4 Short-form McGill Pain Questionnaire
Source: Reproduced with kind permission from Professor Melzeck. Copyright R. Melzack 1975, 1984. Available http://www.npcrc.org/usr_doc/adhoc/painsymptom/McGill%20Pain%20Inventory.pdf

The MPQ comprises a list of 78 words categorised into 20 groups that represent four major dimensions of pain quality: sensory, affective, evaluative and miscellaneous. Each word has a score value, and the patient is asked to select words that describe his or her pain. The short form of the MPQ, illustrated in Figure 2.4, takes less than five minutes to complete and is sensitive to clinical change resulting from pain interventions, for example analgesia (Melzack 1987).

Several scores can be calculated using the MPQ. For example, the total value of the words chosen gives the pain rating index (PRI) for each of the dimensions – sensory, affective, evaluative and miscellaneous. These can also be added together to give the PRI total. The total number of words chosen (NWC) is another score, and there is also the present pain intensity (PPI), which is an intensity score derived from a 0–5 scale. This is a useful tool for gaining a broader perspective of patients' experience of pain and how it is affecting them and is primarily used in chronic pain. For further information regarding these pain assessment tools, see Melzack and Katz (1994).

Brief Pain Inventory

The Brief Pain Inventory (Figure 2.5 below) is another multidimensional pain tool that is particularly useful for specialist pain clinics but would also have utility in general practice for the assessment of chronic pain.

The Leeds Assessment of Neuropathic Symptoms and Signs (LANSS) Pain Scale

The LANSS Pain Scale shown below in Figure 2.6 is an example of a tool that has been developed and validated specifically to help diagnose and assess neuropathic pain. Neuropathic pain is quite different from nociceptive pain and often goes unrecognised. It is characterised by chronic, stimulus-independent pain sensation accompanied by hyperalgesia/allodynia and **paresthesia**. The impact of neuropathic pain can substantially affect the quality of a person's life, which is usefully assessed within the tool. The tool has been used with several different patient groups to identify neuropathic pain including those with cancer (Potter et al. 2003), diabetes (Bennett et al. 2003) and low back pain (Kaki et al. 2005).

Study ID #_____   Hospital #_____

DO NOT WRITE ABOVE THIS LINE

Brief Pain Inventory (Short Form)

Date: _____/_____/_____/   Time: _____

Name: _____   _____   _____
                Last   First   Middle Initial

1. Throughout our lives, most of us have had pain from time to time (such as minor headaches, sprains, and toothaches). Have you had pain other than these everyday kinds of pain today?

1.   Yes   2.   No

2. On the diagram, shade in the areas where you feel pain. Put an X on the area that hurts the most.

3. Please rate your pain by circling the one number that best describes your pain at its worst in the last 24 hours.

   0   1   2   3   4   5   6   7   8   9   10
   No   Pain as bad as
   pain   you can imagine

4. Please rate your pain by circling the one number that best decribes your pain at its least in the last 24 hours.

   0   1   2   3   4   5   6   7   8   9   10
   No   Pain as bad as
   pain   you can imagine

5. Please rate your pain by circling the one number that best decribes your pain on the average.

   0   1   2   3   4   5   6   7   8   9   10
   No   Pain as bad as
   pain   you can imagine

6. Please rate your pain by circling the one number that tells how much pain you have right now.

   0   1   2   3   4   5   6   7   8   9   10
   No   Pain as bad as
   pain   you can imagine

7. What treatments or medications are you receiving for your pain?

8. In the last 24 hours, how much relief have pain treatments or medications provided? Please circle the one percentage that most shows how much relief you have received.

   0%   10%   20%   30%   40%   50%   60%   70%   80%   90%   100%
   No   Complete
   relief   relief

9. Circle the one number that describes how, during the past 24 hours, pain has interfered with your:

A.   General activity

   0   1   2   3   4   5   6   7   8   9   10
   Does not   Completely
   interfere   interferes

B.   Mood

   0   1   2   3   4   5   6   7   8   9   10
   Does not   Completely
   interfere   interferes

C.   Walking ability

   0   1   2   3   4   5   6   7   8   9   10
   Does not   Completely
   interfere   interferes

D.   Normal work (includes both work outside the home and housework)

   0   1   2   3   4   5   6   7   8   9   10
   Does not   Completely
   interfere   interferes

E.   Relations with other people

   0   1   2   3   4   5   6   7   8   9   10
   Does not   Completely
   interfere   interferes

F.   Sleep

   0   1   2   3   4   5   6   7   8   9   10
   Does not   Completely
   interfere   interferes

G.   Enjoyment of life

   0   1   2   3   4   5   6   7   8   9   10
   Does not   Completely
   interfere   interferes

Figure 2.5 The Brief Pain Inventory

Source: Copyright 1991 Charles S. Cleeland, PhD, Pain Research Group. All rights reserved. Used with permission.

Name .... Date ....

LEEDS ASSESSMENT OF NEUROPATHIC SYMPTOMS AND SIGNS

This pain scale can help to determine whether the nerves that are carrying your pain signals are working normally or not. It is important to find this out in case different treatments are needed to control your pain.

A. Pain Questionnaire

☐ Think about how your pain has felt over the last week
☐ Please say whether any of the descriptions match your pain exactly

1) Does your pain feel like strange, unpleasant sensations in your skin? Words like pricking, tingling, pins and needles might describe these sensations.

a) NO – My pain doesn't really feel like this ....(0)
b) YES – I get these sensations quite a lot ....(5)

2) Does your pain make the skin in the painful area look different from normal? Words like mottled or looking more red or pink might describe the appearance.

a) NO – My pain doesn't affect the colour of my skin ....(0)
b) YES – I've noticed that the pain does make my skin look different from normal ....(5)

3) Does your pain make the affected skin abnormally sensitive to touch? Getting unpleasant sensations when lightly stroking the skin, or getting pain when wearing tight clothes might describe the abnormal sensitivity.

a) NO – My pain doesn't make my skin abnormally sensitive in that area ....(0)
b) YES – My skin seems abnormally sensitive to touch in that area ....(3)

4) Does your pain come on suddenly and in bursts for no apparent reason when you're still? Words like electric shocks, jumping and bursting might describe these sensations.

a) NO – My pain doesn't really feel like this ....(0)
b) YES – I get these sensations quite a lot ....(2)

5) Does your pain feel as if the skin temperature in the painful area has changed abnormally? Words like hot and burning might describe these sensations.

a) NO – I don't really get these sensations ....(0)
b) YES – I get these sensations quite a lot ....(1)

Subtotal ☐

Name ....   Date ....

LEEDS ASSESSMENT OF NEUROPATHIC SYMPTOMS AND SIGNS

B. Sensory Testing

Skin sensitivity can be examined by comparing the painful area with a contralateral or adjacent non-painful area for the presence of allodynia and an altered pin-prick threshold (PPT).

1) Allodynia
Examine the response to lightly stroking cotton wool across the non-painful area and the painful area. If normal sensations are experienced in the non-painful site, but pain or unpleasant sensations (tingling, nausea) are experienced in the painful area when stroking, allodynia is present.

a) NO – normal sensation in both areas..(0)
b) YES – allodynia in painful area only ....(5)

2) Altered Pin-prick Threshold
Determine the pin-prick threshold by comparing the response to a 23 gauge (blue) needle mounted inside a 2ml syringe barrel placed gently on to the skin in a non-painful, and then painful area.

If a sharp pin-prick is felt in the non-painful area, but a different sensation is experienced in the painful area eg. none /blunt only (raised PPT) or a very painful sensation (lowered PPT), an altered PPT is present.

If a pin-prick is not felt in either area, mount the syringe onto the needle to increase the weight and repeat.

a) NO – equal sensation in both areas.. .(0)
b) YES – altered PPT in painful area ....(3)

Scoring:

Add values in parentheses for sensory description and examination findings to obtain overall score.

Total score (maximum 24) ....

If score < 12, neuropathic mechanisms are **unlikely** to be contributing to the patient's pain
If score > 12, neuropathic mechanisms are **likely** to be contributing to the patient's pain

Figure 2.6 The LANSS Pain Scale
Source: Bennett (2001) The LANSS Pain Scale: The Leeds Assessment of Neuropathic Symptoms and Signs, *Pain*, **92**: 147–57. Reproduced with kind permission of The International Association for the Study of Pain®

Pain diaries

Asking patients to keep a diary of their pain can be helpful for suffers of chronic pain to gain an understanding of those factors which might exacerbate or reduce their pain. In the community they might be particularly useful and patients often gain benefit from the activity and feel they are participating in their care more fully. Where pain assessment is difficult to incorporate into secondary care, it would be interesting to see how patients perceive their pain control and its evaluation in a diary. One day this sort of assessment may even form part of staff or hospital appraisal. Where diaries have been used for research purposes, however, there has been less success with paper versions compared to electronic ones (Stone et al. 2002). This may be related to the perceived importance of the task.

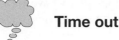 **Time out**

Pain is frequently inadequately assessed. We know that failure to assess pain is a major barrier to its effective control, but few hospitals include pain assessment in their routine patient monitoring. What strategies might encourage practitioners to assess pain? Discuss this with colleagues and see whether you can come up with any suggestions.

Charts for regular everyday use

Getting practice to change is not an easy feat. Pain management and its inadequacies have long been reported, and it has been suggested that one of the reasons why practice has been slow to change is the lack of institutionalised policies that positively affect pain management. In the USA, this is being addressed by making pain assessment mandatory if hospitals are to attain or retain accreditation. The Joint Commission on Accreditation of Healthcare Organizations (JCAHO) lists the following standards for pain and its management (reproduced with permission from JCAHO (2000) *Standards for Pain Assessment and its Management*, JCAHO, Oakbrook Terrace, IL):

- Patients have the right to recognition and control of their pain
- Thorough pain assessment of patients identified with pain
- Perform effective pain management and rehabilitation
- Educate staff, patient and family about pain
- Ongoing quality improvement of pain management.

Figure 2.7 comprises a chart introduced into a district general hospital (DGH) some years ago to encourage the routine and regular assessment of acute pain. Although it is fairly straightforward, its use was sporadic and unsatisfactory. The assessment tool in Figure 2.7 is located in the lower portion of the standard observation chart for temperature, pulse and blood pressure. A pain score is charted in the special boxed section. The boxes are divided in two by a diagonal line. Should a patient report moderate or severe pain, this is scored in the top section of the box and indicated by the letter P. Analgesia is then administered, and the patient's pain is reassessed within the hour. The repeat score is then charted in the bottom half of the box. If a strong opioid is administered, the chart enables the sedation score also to be documented in the bottom half of the box. The development of this chart was part of a hospital-wide policy to raise the profile of pain management and incorporate an 'institutionalised' practice to encourage nurses regularly to monitor and document pain assessment. However, it proved to be a complete failure. Figure 2.8 represents a chart currently in use at the same DGH that appears to have gained greater acceptance. It is simple and easy to complete and can convey a considerable amount of information.

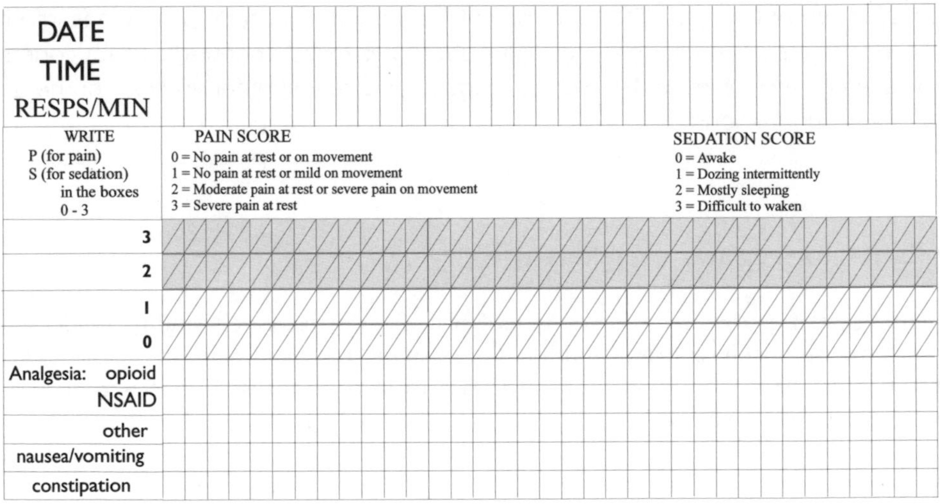

Figure 2.7 Chart for recording acute pain intensity

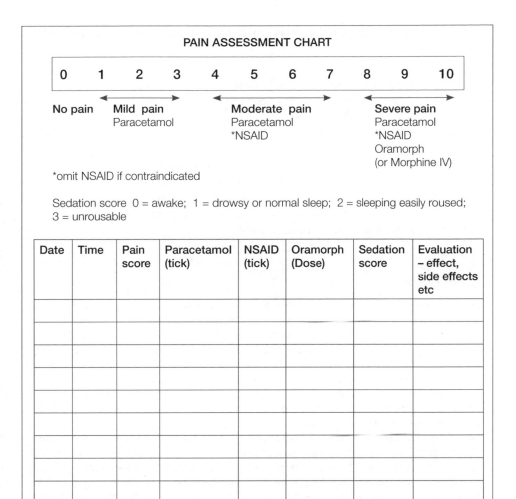

Figure 2.8 Acute pain assessment chart
Source: By kind permission of Poole Hospital NHS Trust

It would seem that nurses still assume that patients will tell them when they are in pain, although this rarely happens in reality. Most patients expect the nurse to know that they are in pain and to enquire about their pain, so we are left with a fundamental communication barrier that can prove difficult to remove (Franke and Theeuwen 1994). The motivation to assess and manage pain more effectively can be influenced by how the organisation in which pain management takes place views pain. Recent work has drawn on the aviation industry and put pain management in the category of 'patient safety' (Leape et al. 2002). This can change the way an organisation responds and is discussed further in Chapter 7.

Charts to monitor continuous epidural and patient controlled analgesia

As we have moved to more 'high-tech' pain management strategies, so there has been a need to develop specific assessment tools to ensure that these can be safely managed on general wards.

Patient controlled analgesia (PCA) enables powerful drugs to be administered directly into the bloodstream, while continuous or patient controlled epidural analgesia enables medication access into the epidural space in the spine of patients. Although these strategies will be covered in more detail in Chapter 4, Figure 2.9 is an example of an epidural pain assessment chart that incorporates the prescription of boluses (regular doses) and top-ups (from the bag of epidural solution) combined with a monitoring and maintenance protocol.

Case history

Mrs King was admitted to the ward following major bowel surgery with a low thoracic epidural in place. She was comfortable; monitoring was acceptable including normal sensation. The only thing Mrs King commented on was that she was having a bit of trouble moving her legs. This was documented on a regular basis but nothing was mentioned to the acute pain team or senior medical staff as it was assumed that as the epidural was reduced, leg mobility would return. Unfortunately, several hours had passed before she was assessed by the acute pain team, who noted normal sensation but by then almost complete loss of lower limb function. Medical assistance was immediately requested. During the immediate postoperative period, Mrs King had experienced several periods of hypotension. Although this was acted on following the protocols in place, the workload on the ward at the time meant there had been a short delay in restoring satisfactory blood pressure. It transpired that Mrs King had experienced a spinal infarct possibly during one of these periods of hypotension. This may not have been avoidable but an early response to her reducing limb function while sensation remained intact should have rung alarm bells much sooner. Mrs King did go on to recover some mobility but was left with a handicap.

This highlights the need to provide continuous education for ward staff to ensure they remain vigilant for the onset of problems.

Epidural Analgesia Prescription

Addressograph	Consultant surgeon Ward Dare Anaesthetist

EPIDURAL SOLUTION

Date	Solution	Infusion rate	Signature
	Bupivicaine 0.125 % + Fentanyl 4mcg in sodium chloride 0.9% in 500 ml	2–	SIGN ONE
	Bupivicaine 0.1 % + Fentanyl 2mcg in sodium chloride 0.9% in 500 ml	2–	OF THESE
	Bupivicaine 0.15 % in Sodium chloride 0.9% in 500 ml	2–	BOXES
	3ml bolus x 3 of epidural solution <u>authorised staff only</u> PIRITON 4 mg P.O. or NALOXONE 0.2 mg I.M for itching GELOFUSINE 500 mls stat if systolic BP < 80 mmhg		SIGN THIS BOX

EXTRA INFUSIONS

Date	Time	Infusion	Signature

BOLUS/TOP-UPS

Date	Time	Solution	Volume	Signature

MONITORING AND MAINTENANCE FOR PATIENT RECEIVING EPIDURAL

Observation	Action
Respiratory rate	If respiratory rate is <10/min stop the pump If respiratory rate is <8 stop pump and inform P3
Blood pressure	If systolic BP is <80 mmhg give Gelofusine 500 mls stat
Pain intensity 0 = No pain at rest or on movement 1–4 = No pain at rest or mild pain on movement 5–7 = Moderate pain at rest, severe on moving 8–10 = Severe pain at rest	Pain intensity 1–4 give Paracetamol/NSAID if appropriate 5–7 as above and increase epidural infusion 8–10 increase rate and inform APS (P3 out of hours)
Sedation score 0 = Alert patient/normal sleep (rousable) 1 = Mild (occasionally drowsy, rousable) 2 = Moderate (frequently drowsy, easily roused) 3 = Severe (somnolent, difficult to rouse)	If patient is unrousable, stop epidural infusion and inform P3
Sensation 0 = Normal sensation 1 = Altered sensation (to touch or temperature) 2 = Absence of sensation	If there is any altered sensation of legs (or arms) call APS (P3 out of hours)
Motor power 0 = Normal power 1 = Weakness but can lift against gravity 2 = Cannot move limb against gravity 3 = Cannot move limb	If there is any limb motor weakness call APS (P3 out of hours)
Pruritus (itching) 0 = No pruritus 1 = pruritus 2 = uncomfortable	Administer piriton 4 mg po as first line treatment If no response, consider Naloxone 0.2 mg IM

Observations must be recorded:
- Half hourly for 2 hours
- Hourly for 4 hours
- Four hourly thereafter

Date	Time	Rate ml/hr	Total infused	Pain at rest	Pain on movement	Sedation score	Resp rate	Blood pressure	Sensory score L	R	Motor score L	R	Site checked	Comments signature

Date epidural discontinued ....

Nurse removing epidural ....

Signs of infection: YES/NO

Tip/Swab sent for culture YES/NO

Figure 2.9 Epidural pain assessment and monitoring chart
Source: By kind permission of Poole Hospital NHS Trust

Changing practice: introducing a pain assessment tool

Selecting a pain assessment tool for use in clinical practice requires careful consideration as well as an appreciation of the potential for error, as the interpretation of data from a pain rating scale is not as straightforward as it might first appear (Williamson and Hoggart 2005). Mackintosh (2007) discusses assessment and management of postoperative pain, while Karoly et al. (2006) give a little insight into the challenges of chronic pain assessment in the community. See whether any of the tools reviewed seem particularly useful for your clinical area and then complete the activity.

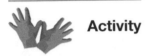 **Activity**

Choose one pain assessment tool that you feel would be appropriate for your client group. Assess the pain of 5–10 clients (you might want to modify the tool a little).

When assessing their pain, consider how 'good' the tool is at accurately identifying the level and type of pain. Make notes about how easy the tool was to use, how long it took to administer and what your patients felt about you using the tool. Did you get any surprises? Think about the patient you interviewed at the start of this chapter. How did the information differ when you were assessing pain with a formal tool compared to when you asked casual questions?

You have probably found out from your various activities that, for acute pain, you need a simple tool to assess the site of the pain and its intensity. As chronic pain has such an adverse impact on the quality of life, far more information is usually incorporated into the chart. Not only are site and intensity important, but other factors could also be particularly significant. We need to know what the pain feels like and how often it occurs. Is it there constantly? What are the aggravating or relieving factors? What is the duration of the pain? How does the pain affect the way a patient feels, and what impact does the pain have on a patient's quality of life, sleep, mobility and many other factors? A tool that enables the documentation of all the strategies that are helpful, both pharmacological and non-pharmacological, will lead to good communication and ensure that previously unhelpful strategies are not reintroduced.

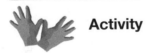 **Activity**

For some people who live with chronic pain day in, day out, assessing their pain regularly might be detrimental. Why is this, and what could you do to ensure that assessment did not result in a worsening of their ability to cope with their pain?

People experiencing chronic pain often use strategies such as distraction to mini-mise their pain; regular questions about their pain may, however, reduce the effec-tiveness of this distraction. With chronic pain, especially when a cure is unlikely, assessment may take place on a daily, weekly or even less frequent basis. New treat-ments or therapies will need fairly frequent evaluation, but regularly making a patient refocus on his or her chronic pain could be counterproductive.

Conclusion

Pain assessment and documentation is essential for the effective management of pain. Interestingly, although nurses may have good intentions about completing documenta-tion and assessment charts, research continues to reveal their failure to do so. This chapter has explored the process of pain assessment and considered not only factors that can affect an individual's perception and expression of pain, but also pain assessment tools that can be utilised in clinical practice. Convincing practitioners of the importance of pain assessment tools can be a difficult process, yet it is of paramount importance that pain assessment is incorporated into daily practice, whether it be in hospital or in a community setting. Bias, stereotyping and the inaccurate collection of information can all contribute to errors in assessment and the ongoing utilisation of inadequate or inap-propriate pain management (Gunningberg and Idvall 2007). An accurate, sensitive and detailed assessment forms the foundation of effective management.

The following statement introduces 'a new pain manifesto' to make pain the fifth vital sign (Hall 2005) in the UK:

> If pain were routinely assessed with the same priority as blood pressure, pulse, respiration and temperature, then a great deal of unnecessary suffering, stress and anxiety could be avoided.

To conclude, you might like to try and memorise this simple mnemonic – ABCDE:

Ask about pain regularly; assess pain systematically
Believe the patient and family in their reports of pain and what relieves it
Choose pain control options appropriate for the patient, family and setting
Deliver interventions in a timely, logical and coordinated fashion
Empower patients and their families; enable them to take control to the greatest extent possible (Jacox et al.1994).

After a break, try the multiple choice test below in order to self-assess your understanding so far. For some of the questions, more than one answer will be correct, however, there will be one answer that is best supported by the evidence.

Suggested further reading

Sjostrom B., Dahlgren L. and Haljame H. (2000) Strategies used in post-operative pain assessment and their clinical accuracy. *Journal of Clinical Nursing*, **9**: 111–18.

Sloman R., Rosen G., Rom M. and Shir Y. (2004) Nurses' assessment of pain in surgical patients. *Journal of Advanced Nursing,* **52**(2): 125–32.

Mackintosh C. (2007) Assessment and management of patients with post-operative pain. *Nursing Standard*, 22(5): 49–55.

Turk D. and Melzack R. (eds) (2001) *Handbook of Pain Assessment*, 2nd edn. New York, Guildford Press.

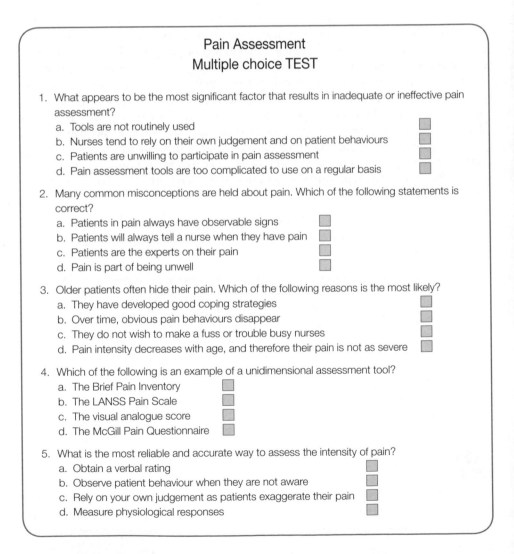

Pain Assessment
Multiple choice TEST

1. What appears to be the most significant factor that results in inadequate or ineffective pain assessment?
    a. Tools are not routinely used
    b. Nurses tend to rely on their own judgement and on patient behaviours
    c. Patients are unwilling to participate in pain assessment
    d. Pain assessment tools are too complicated to use on a regular basis

2. Many common misconceptions are held about pain. Which of the following statements is correct?
    a. Patients in pain always have observable signs
    b. Patients will always tell a nurse when they have pain
    c. Patients are the experts on their pain
    d. Pain is part of being unwell

3. Older patients often hide their pain. Which of the following reasons is the most likely?
    a. They have developed good coping strategies
    b. Over time, obvious pain behaviours disappear
    c. They do not wish to make a fuss or trouble busy nurses
    d. Pain intensity decreases with age, and therefore their pain is not as severe

4. Which of the following is an example of a unidimensional assessment tool?
    a. The Brief Pain Inventory
    b. The LANSS Pain Scale
    c. The visual analogue score
    d. The McGill Pain Questionnaire

5. What is the most reliable and accurate way to assess the intensity of pain?
    a. Obtain a verbal rating
    b. Observe patient behaviour when they are not aware
    c. Rely on your own judgement as patients exaggerate their pain
    d. Measure physiological responses

6. Which pain assessment tool is the most effective for the measurement of small changes in pain intensity?
   a. A verbal rating scale ☐
   b. A visual analogue scale ☐
   c. A 'faces' rating scale ☐
   d. A 0–10 numerical rating scale ☐

7. How many scores can be calculated for the McGill Pain Questionnaire?
   a. Two ☐
   b Seven ☐
   c. Four ☐
   d. Three ☐

8. Which activity would be most likely to improve effective pain assessment?
   a. Asking patients to complete their own assessment charts ☐
   b. Institutionalising pain assessment – making it a hospital policy to regularly assess and document pain ☐
   c. Regular visits by pain teams ☐
   d. More time ☐

9. If someone is experiencing chronic pain, why might frequent pain assessment be detrimental?
   a. It is too time-consuming ☐
   b. By focusing on the pain, it risks compromising patients' coping strategies ☐
   c. It encourages patients to exaggerate their pain ☐
   d. There is little that can be done to manage chronic pain so there is little point ☐

10. To complement the data collected by a verbal rating pain assessment tool, what other information might be the next most useful?
    a. Blood pressure, pulse rate and respiratory rate ☐
    b. A medical and family history ☐
    c. Any previous experience of pain, and the coping strategies used ☐
    d. Observation of the patient's behaviour ☐

Answers

1. b. Nurses rely on their own judgement and on patient behaviour; evidence suggests that nurses do not use formal assessment tools that would help patients to communicate a subjective experience. Instead, they rely on their own judgement and patients' behaviour. If a patient is not demonstrating overt 'pain behaviour' (for example grimacing or becoming withdrawn), nurses may wrongly assume that they are not experiencing pain. The introduction of pain assessment tools is obviously a major factor but research suggests that even when these are in place, they are rarely completed on a regular basis. Patients are usually quite keen to participate in pain assessment and the tools do not need to be complicated.

2. c. Patients are the experts on their pain; patients should not expect to have pain while in hospital, although unfortunately many do. Observable signs of pain are extremely unreliable, and a large number of patients will not report when they are in pain: they will expect the nurse to know about their pain. Pain should not be part of illness unless this is acceptable to a patient.

3. c. Older people are often reluctant to trouble 'busy' nurses and can become very accepting of pain. Although they may well develop coping strategies, this is not usually given as a reason. There is no compelling evidence that pain intensity decreases with age, and that therefore older people's pain is not as severe or that pain behaviour decreases over time.

4. c. The visual analogue score; all the others assess a wide range of responses to pain and the effect pain has on a sufferer.

5. a. Obtain a verbal rating. Only the patient knows how bad their pain is.

6. b. A visual analogue scale will provide the greatest sensitivity when it comes to measuring pain intensity. Verbal ratings are good for determining the quality of the pain but usually only have a maximum of five words. Likewise 'faces' rating scales usually only include six progressive levels. A numerical rating of 0–10 increases choice but the visual analogue usually has a measure of 0–100 on the reverse side of a 10 cm line.

7. c. Seven, comprising the total value of the words from the four dimensions (sensory, affective, evaluative and miscellaneous) which can be added together to give the PRI total, the total number of words chosen and the PPI.

8. a. Although this is a rather difficult question, encouraging patients to complete their own pain assessment charts may well prove to be the most effective. Introducing institution-wide pain assessment and linking it to accreditation, as has happened in the USA, has not thus far been quite as effective as one would expect. Although an increased number of visits from the pain team might be beneficial, it might also reduce the ward nurses' perceived responsibility for pain management. More time is often cited as a reason for less than optimum pain management but there is no evidence that providing more staff and time necessarily have a positive impact on pain management.

9. b. By focusing on the pain, it reduces patients' coping strategies. When someone is using distraction to take their mind off pain, frequent assessments can negatively impact on this coping strategy and cause them to focus on their pain again. Regular pain assessment need not be time-consuming, especially if patients are encouraged to participate in the process. It is unlikely that they will exaggerate their pain: they are in fact more likely to minimise it. There are many interventions for chronic pain that have been shown to help people to cope with their pain.

10. c. Any previous experience of pain, and the coping strategies used; ascertaining these is invaluable in gaining a better understanding of the meaning of pain for this person and how best to incorporate previous interventions that have been helpful. Physiological and behavioural observations are notoriously unreliable. The medical and family history may or may not be directly related to the current pain experience. In addition, people may experience pain when there is no evident pathology.

CHAPTER 3

Recognising the Barriers to Effective Pain Relief

Learning outcomes

On completion of this chapter, the student will be able to:

- Critically discuss the effects of the inadequate knowledge and inappropriate attitudes of healthcare professionals on the management of pain

- Identify factors that contribute to patients' minimising their pain, and strategies that might reduce their impact

- Evaluate organisational policies and practices that might contribute to ineffective pain management

- Understand how political influences can exert a negative impact on pain management

Indicative reading

Brockopp D., Brockopp G., Warden S., Wilson J., Carpenter J. et al. (1998) Barrier to change: a pain management project. *International Journal of Nursing Studies*, **35**: 226–32.

Carr E.C.J. (2007) Barriers to effective pain management in perioperative care. *Journal of Perioperative Care*, **17**(5): 200–3, 206–7.

Duignan M. and Dunn V. (2008) Barriers to pain management in emergency departments. *Emergency Nursing*, **15**(9): 30–4.

Glajchen M. (2001) Chronic pain: treatment barriers and strategies for clinical practice. *Journal of American Board of Family Practitioners*, **14**(3): 178–83, http://www.medscape.com/viewpublication/67.

Jacobsen R., Sjøgren P., Møldrup C. and Christrup L. (2007) Physician-related barriers to cancer pain management with opioid analgesics: a systematic review. *Journal of Opioid Management*, **3**(4): 207–14.

Paice J., Barnard C., Creamer J. and Omerod K. (2006) Creating organizational change through the Pain Resource Nurse program. *Joint Commission Journal on Quality and Patient Safety*, **32**(1): 24–31.

Wilson B. (2007) Nurses' knowledge of pain. *Journal of Clinical Nursing*, **16**(6): 1012–20.

Background

Effective pain control is a contemporary issue of immense importance because of the devastating and dehumanising effects it can have upon an individual. Pain indiscriminately crosses age and client groups. The focus of this chapter is primarily on the barriers to effective pain management that can be posed by the attitudes, knowledge, policies and practices of healthcare professionals, patients, their carers and organisations. The management of pain in vulnerable and challenging patient groups may create additional and unique demands/barriers, which are discussed in more detail in Chapters 6 and 7.

Nursing the patient who is experiencing pain requires contemporary knowledge, skilled interventions (both pharmacological and non-pharmacological) and attitudes that convey trust, empathy and an honest belief in the patient. This may seem simple, yet the real world presents daily complexities and challenges that confront the clinicians who manage pain. This chapter covers some well-documented 'barriers' to effective pain management and outlines appropriate strategies in an attempt to lessen their impact. In reflecting on your own clinical practice and a sense of having 'been there', recognising these barriers can be frustrating. However, we hope that this chapter will enthuse, motivate and invite you to feel more confident in contributing to effective pain management.

Healthcare professionals

In the early 1990s, when inadequate pain management was first recognised on a wide scale, Griepp (1992) reviewed 15 pain studies and identified the 'knowledge deficit' of professionals as being the most prevalent reason for inadequate pain management. Since then, literature on the barriers to pain management has flourished and undoubtedly pain education has improved, with the results of later knowledge surveys suggesting some benefit (McCaffrey and Ferrell 1997) but perhaps not as much as you would expect. Despite some improvement, the bottom line is that even in the area of postoperative pain, arguably the most straightforward pain encountered, inadequate management of pain is common, with over three-quarters of patients sampled reporting moderate, severe or extreme pain (Apfelbaum et al. 2003) and lack of knowledge still given as a concern.

Although effective analgesic techniques are available, they are frequently not used. The reasons for this have been attributed to physicians' failure to prescribe effective analgesia and their adherence to dosage schedules known to be ineffective, as well as to the inappropriate attitudes and beliefs of both nurses and doctors (McCaffery et al. 1990; Clarke et al. 1996). Studies expanding on these conclusions reveal more subtle barriers to improving pain practice that we explore within this chapter.

Nurses are not the only ones who have been found to have a deficiency in their pain knowledge. A survey of 27 medical schools revealed that four undertook no formal teaching on pain control, while the remainder averaged only 3.5 hours during a five-year course (Marcer and Deighton 1988). It is worrying that this important work is now quite dated and yet it has not been replicated in the UK. A recent survey of students undertaking veterinary and health science degrees in Canada revealed that those undertaking veterinary degrees received over three times as many hours on specific pain education than doctors, nurses, physiotherapists, dentists and other healthcare professionals (Watt-Watson et al. 2007).

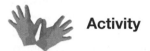 **Activity**

Find three research articles on 'pain and education'. What were the researchers trying to find out? What methods did they use to answer the research question(s)?

Most researchers are trying to assess the knowledge and attitudes of healthcare professionals. The usual method for doing this is a questionnaire. Questionnaires can be helpful to measure how much people know about a subject, but do not tell you whether they use this knowledge in their practice. Someone filling in the questionnaire may give all the right answers but not have the confidence to use the knowledge in practice. Research using other methods such as observation and measuring patient outcomes gives more insightful answers (Schafheutle et al. 2001). It would be logical to expect that practitioners with a high level of pain knowledge would give better care (as patients experienced less pain) than practitioners with less knowledge. A literature review of nurse education found that despite extensive postoperative pain education programmes, nurses did not necessarily comply with medication orders, seemingly confirming that improved knowledge alone may not be sufficient to enhance pain management (Wilson 2007).

These are some examples of the common misconceptions surrounding pain that are held by practitioners and reported in research studies:

- Patients should expect pain in hospital
- Obvious pathology, abnormal test results and the type of surgery determine the existence and intensity of pain
- Patients in pain always have observable signs
- Chronic pain is not as serious as acute pain
- Patients will always tell you when they have pain
- One type of pain intervention, for example analgesia, is sufficient to relieve pain
- Addiction and respiratory depression are major problems with opioid use
- Patients should have pain before being given analgesia
- Patients who laugh and chat to visitors cannot have that much pain
- Patients will exaggerate their pain and should not always be believed.

In addition to the above misconceptions, the seminal work by Fagerhaugh and Strauss in 1977 asserted that patients have been subtly encouraged to conform to health professionals' expectations. Although we would assume this is no longer the case, later work by Clements and Cummings (1991) demonstrated that patients who did not conform to staff expectations were perceived by nurses as manipulative and demanding in relation to their pain management. It has also been mooted that staff can become desensitised to pain (Blomquist and Edberg 2002). Wilson (2007) suggests that inadequacies in pain management may not just be tied to misconception, myth, bias and inadequate knowledge but to how increased knowledge is applied. Her work studies the influence of the working environment on the development and implementation of knowledge by nurses, implying that it is the work environment that can induce feelings of reduced self-efficacy and low personal control. This suggests that nurses, given the knowledge but not encouraged to implement it in practice, risk becoming demoralised. To ease tension, they may refuse to endorse their knowledge. It is no good knowing how to do things better if you perceive yourself as powerless to make the decisions and implement real change, which will happen if nurses feel hampered by a lack of supportive consultation between colleagues and a pressure to conform to the prevailing 'norms'.

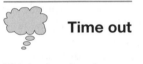

Time out

Think about pain management in your clinical area. Do any of the above statements ring true? Why do you think these views are held?

The effective management of pain relies on the teamwork of different professionals, each with a valuable contribution. As already mentioned, it is essential that they have the appropriate knowledge to manage pain effectively. Even more important is the ability to work together and communicate effectively, yet conflict and misunderstanding can make working as a team difficult (Brockopp et al. 1998).

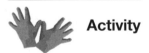

Activity

Think of a patient you have cared for who has experienced pain. Reflect on the role of the different professionals involved in that person's care. Was there any difficulty or conflict between the professionals, or between the patient and a professional?

Communication between professionals is not always as clear as it could be. A nurse might identify a patient who is experiencing a lot of pain and ask the doctor to change the analgesic prescription. The doctor might find that the patient does not appear to have much pain and think that the analgesia prescription is adequate.

Conflict can occur when the nurse washes the patient and finds that turning him causes pain and distress. If the doctor and nurse had discussed this person's pain together (with the patient), this might not have happened. Many doctors are uncomfortable when confronted with patients in pain as they lack the training to feel confident in their prescribing (O'Rouke 2007). The nurse may in fact be far more knowledgeable on pain and analgesia and this would have been conveyed if they were working well together as a team. Bringing different professions together to discuss and learn about pain management can improve communication in the clinical area, which ultimately facilitates improved pain management (Carr et al. 2003). There has been considerable focus on the use of interprofessional pain education in practice.

Improving practice

Case history

The nurses in a small palliative care team were expressing their frustration at trying to manage a patient's pain that was not responding to the prescribed analgesia. The patient was having to wait a considerable time as the doctor was busy in A&E on the other side of the hospital. The doctors and nurses discussed possible solutions to the problem and came up with the idea of ensuring that pain was assessed before 8 a.m. A protocol was drawn up to cover the administration of 'one-off' analgesia in certain situations, and a list of non-pharmacological strategies that could be utilised to help the patient in the interim period. The discussion led the nurses to reflect on how pain was currently assessed and managed. They realised that if a patient's pain had been closely monitored, it was unlikely that this situation would occur at all.

The simplest of strategies can be the most effective and often arise when just a few interested professionals manage to take the time to discuss what could be improved and how to improve it.

The inadequate knowledge of healthcare professionals remains a prevalent causative factor in studies documenting the undertreatment of pain (Clarke et al. 1996; Glajchen and Bookbinder 2001). The majority of nurse education undergraduate programmes include pain management in the curriculum, but clearly this is insufficient to counter the considerable fear and ignorance particularly relating to opioids (Cowan et al. 2003, 2004). As previously mentioned, Marcer and Deighton (1988) originally highlighted the problem of little or no pain education for medical students, with scant evidence of multidisciplinary teaching. Despite an increasing emphasis being placed on the need to improve pain education for medical staff, many qualified doctors still feel ill prepared (O'Rorke 2007) and serious deficits in the knowledge of medical students persist (Lasch et al. 2002).

Funnell (1995) reviewed the literature and identified four expected outcomes associated with shared learning. Understanding the roles and perceptions of other professionals, and the promotion of future teamwork, leads to cooperation between professional groups. This in turn contributes to enhancing the learner's knowledge base and the development of practical skills.

The term 'interprofessional' suggests shared learning, which aims to help professionals to work together more effectively. Interprofessional education has been defined as 'Occasions when two or more professions learn from and about each other to improve collaboration and the quality of care' (CAIPE 1997). Interprofessional pain education should explicitly link to the everyday world of clinical practice; for example, if the prescribed analgesia is not relieving the pain, the nurse needs the knowledge and skills to negotiate a change in the prescription. Education must address the knowledge, skills and confidence required to deliver effective pain management in a multiprofessional environment.

A questionnaire was given to all teachers in Finnish medical faculties in 1991 and 1995 (Poyhia and Kalso 1999), using the International Association for the Study of Pain (IASP) curricula to evaluate and compare with current teaching. The results were disappointing, revealing no printed curriculum in any university, and the picture had not changed between 1991 and 1995. A serious lack of time allotted to the psychology of pain was found within the teaching. Recommendations were made to focus on changing the attitudes of the university teachers to pain, including that the IASP should distribute curricula to the governing bodies of the universities and that a multimedia teaching package be produced to accompany the curricula.

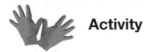 **Activity**

How could you promote interprofessional pain education in your practice?

A study day with breakout sessions and smaller group workshops would be one way of providing an opportunity for different professionals to come together and learn about pain, but time constraints and resources are often prohibitive. It might be possible to build pain education into some activities that already involve different professionals coming together, for example a case conference or ward round. Having 15 minutes to discuss a particular patient and his or her pain management can encourage professionals to share their viewpoints and problem-solve. Alternatively, sharing a research paper and discussing it informally can get people thinking differently about pain management in their clinical area. Although it is generally agreed that the way forward is interprofessional education, the evidence so far has not been particularly helpful in determining the best way to actually achieve this (Irajpour 2006), so there is plenty of room for improvement.

Case history

Pilkington Ward is a busy adult oncology ward. A recent pain audit revealed that many patients experienced unrelieved pain. When the ward staff received the feedback from the audit, they were rather dismayed as they thought that they had been quite good with pain control. One nurse said: 'Well, we do our best, but the problem is that the patients refuse analgesia when it is offered.' Using a problem-solving approach, the ward team decided to conduct a small improvement project on 'patients refusing analgesia'.

Identifying the problem: how many patients refuse analgesia and why?
A sheet of paper was taped to the inside of the drug trolley, nurses noting down when patients were asked whether they would like analgesia and what their response was (acceptance or refusal):

- If patients refused analgesia, they were asked why.
- Of all the patients who were asked whether they would like an analgesic, 70% refused.
- Most patients preferred not to take analgesia, would wait until later or did not have pain.

Making some small changes
Many patients did not see that good pain relief was important or they preferred to tolerate the pain rather than endure the unpleasant side effects of analgesia (such as constipation). Some patients believed that pain could not be relieved or that medication was not an effective way to control pain. Many had a strong belief that addiction and tolerance would become a problem. Some feared that medications taken now would not be effective in the future when they really needed them. Interestingly, in a study of patients receiving chemotherapy, concerns were voiced that expressing pain might distract doctors from treating the underlying disease and that 'good patients' do not complain about their pain.

It also became apparent that not all nurses asked patients about their pain in the same way, and that there was a lack of pain assessment. The team got together and decided to make three small changes in an attempt to encourage patients to accept analgesia when offered:

- On each drug round, the nurse would ask patients to score their pain on a 0–10 scale, which would then be noted on the TPR chart. This would enable nurses to evaluate the effectiveness of previous analgesia and encourage patients to accept analgesia based on their previous pain score.
- A patient information sheet on analgesia was designed. This included why it was important to be comfortable to move, how to manage side effects and what to do if pain relief was not effective. This sheet was given to all patients at the preadmission clinic and on admission to the ward.
- To meet the education needs of the nurses on the ward, a 'tip of the week' was created, which could be a couple of sentences about the key findings from a piece of research, with the reference. This was laminated and taped to the inside of the drug trolley.

Evaluating the effectiveness
After six months, a re-audit revealed that only 58% of patients refused analgesia. This was positive feedback and encouraged the nurses to look at other ways in which they might continue to reduce the number of patients refusing analgesia. (This is based on a real project, published by Carr in 2002.)

This approach, where the problem is identified and followed by a cycle of activities around a model of 'plan-do-study-act', is known as 'quality improvement' (Berwick 1998). It is simple to use and an exciting way of improving the delivery of healthcare. Several good projects have been conducted around the experiences of people in pain and are well worth reading (Gordon et al. 2002).

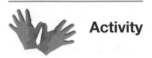 **Activity**

Design a short questionnaire to give to your own professional group. Ideally, this should take no more than 10 minutes to complete. Ask a few questions about their knowledge of and attitudes towards pain.
For example:

- How would you define pain?
- What is the chance of someone becoming addicted to morphine if they receive regular opioids, for trauma, over a two-week period?
  - 30%
  - Less than 1%
  - 60%
  - Don't know

When you have collected this information, try to summarise your findings; putting the answers into a table format can help. Then write up your findings and the implications of your survey in relation to the management of patients' pain. Reflect on the process of this activity. How did you feel about carrying out the survey and the information you found?

Obtaining information from your own practice area, or seeing what is happening elsewhere, can be interesting and informative. It may act as a catalyst for conversations between colleagues and for suggestions on improving practice. It can also raise the awareness of a particular problem or issue. If the findings are not very good or give rise for concern, there may be feelings of guilt or anxiety to do something. Clinical supervision may offer an opportunity to discuss these feelings and offer support to implement some badly needed changes.

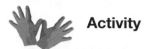

Activity

Now go back and read some of those articles on healthcare professionals' knowledge and attitudes in relation to pain. Compare your findings with those written in the literature. What do you find?

You will have found, through your own reading, that a lack of knowledge and the inappropriate attitudes of healthcare professionals remain two of the major contributions to the ineffective management of patients' pain but many more are surfacing. Did your findings bear any similarity to those of other research in the area? It is clear from the studies emerging that education programmes alone will not change this status quo. It is depressing that over 30 years have elapsed since the work of Fagerhaugh and Strauss revealed inadequacies in professionals' understanding of pain management. A comprehensive programme of undergraduate pain education, which enables different professional groups to come together and learn about pain management, is certainly an important starting point (Watt-Watson et al. 2004), but education must continue after college or university, with regular opportunities for colleagues to come together and share learning. This is particularly important for nurses who wish to specialise in pain management, as concerns have been raised as to whether they can currently access appropriate education for the roles that they undertake (Williamson-Smith 2007).

Patient barriers to effective pain management

Effective pain management can be challenging when patients are unable or have difficulty in communicating their pain, for example small children, neonates, people with learning disabilities and those whose culture is different from that of the healthcare professional. These issues are given greater consideration in Chapters 6 and 7. We now consider some of the everyday reasons why patients may minimise their pain. Despite the best will in the world, there are times when patients are reluctant to report their pain to nurses or doctors (Brockopp et al. 1998). There are several reasons why this may happen, even when we may have emphasised how important it is that they tell us about their pain.

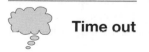

Time out

Think about why patients are likely not to report their pain to you. Make a list of possible reasons.

Some common attitudes and misconceptions about pain from a patient's perspective are:

- Pain is to be expected following surgery, because of disease or cancer
- I have no control over my pain
- Opioids cause too many problems, for example constipation, sickness, sleepiness and addiction
- Constipation from pain medication cannot be relieved
- Pain medication can damage your immune system
- Pain medication makes you do and say embarrassing things
- I don't like putting 'rubbish' in my body
- Pain medication is unnatural and can be dangerous
- I don't want to do some damage because painkillers masked the problem
- I prefer to grin and bear pain
- People are too soft, they should not make a fuss
- Using analgesia is a sign of weakness
- I am quite good at dealing with pain
- I should wait as long as possible before taking a painkiller
- The nurse knows whether I need a painkiller or not
- The nurses are too busy for me to ask for a painkiller
- If I need a higher dose of a strong painkiller, I am becoming an addict
- I can only have painkillers for my pain and I would prefer not to.

Minimising pain is a very real problem for some patients (and their carers), which can impede genuine attempts to manage their pain effectively. To date, there have been relatively few studies exploring the patient's contribution to pain management. Many of the medical research studies assume patients to be the passive recipients of their treatment, and Reisner (1993) argues that the views of the patient have been eclipsed in medicine. This may be changing with the advent of the ethics movement and greater interest in outcomes as we try to move the views of the patients to the centre of healthcare.

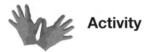 **Activity**

Ask a few patients who they see as being the authority on their pain. In light of their comments, is there anything you would do differently?

We explore some common reasons for patient's minimising their pain in a little more depth.

Patients think the nurse is the authority on their pain

If patients view you as the one who knows most about their pain, they are unlikely to share their true feelings with you; they may assume that you will know when they need analgesia. This could be further endorsed if a general question such as 'Have you any pain Mr Brown?' is asked during the drug round. Patients may assume that the nurse knows whether they need analgesia so they are likely to refuse any unless they feel that the nurse thinks they should have some. In some situations, for example after surgery, it may be more helpful for the nurse to assume that the patient will have some pain or discomfort. Letting patients know that you expect them to have pain/ discomfort may help them to tell you more about their pain. It is important to combine this with a formal pain assessment. (Refer back to Chapter 2 for examples of simple assessment tools.)

Low expectations about pain relief

Scott and Hodson (1997) surveyed 529 people attending their GP about their knowledge of postoperative pain and the methods available to treat it. They found that the public had confidence in the ability of the doctors and nurses to treat this pain and little understanding of postoperative pain or the methods available to control pain. In perioperative care, a study investigating patients' knowledge of common medical terms and their surgical care revealed that many held misconceptions about pain management and a significant number were unaware that the anaesthetist was medically qualified (Laffey et al. 2000). It is essential that we educate patients with regard to their pain relief, otherwise they will continue to have low expectations, which will only serve to perpetuate poor standards (Svenssen et al. 2001).

Culture and religion

A variety of cultural and religious beliefs and attitudes may also serve as a barrier. Middleton (2004) suggests that it may be more acceptable in certain cultures for women to verbalise expressions of pain but for men this would be seen as a sign of weakness. A study exploring the cancer pain experience of Hispanic patients living in the USA revealed that traditional gender roles, cultural values and marginalised status as immigrants influenced the ability of these people to describe and manage their pain (Im et al. 2007). In the UK, the cultural norm regarding pain has been one of endurance and just get on with it – the British 'stiff upper lip'. This attitude can be combined with a common cultural belief that drugs should be used as little as possible (Townsend et al. 2003). There is a sense of pride in showing stoicism, which has been admired and rewarded (Harper et al. 2007). Christian beliefs may leave patients feeling that pain is God's will and must be endured. Surprisingly, this view may be supported by some doctors who are reluctant to prescribe opioids even for cancer patients unless pain is very severe, believing that suffering is a valuable part of human existence (Brockopp et al. 1998).

Fear of injections

In children, the fear of needles is recognised, and the regular use of topical local anaesthetics, as well as the greater use of intravenous, intranasal and oral medication has largely overcome the problem. Integrating calming techniques, structuring the environment and fostering a culture of empathy and respect have been found to be helpful (Ives 2007). In the adult population, this fear is largely ignored, yet many adults also fear injections. Sensitive assessment should identify individuals who fear needles, although it can be powerfully argued that this route of administration is now obsolete and unnecessary. When a patient cannot tolerate oral medications, an intravenous line will be required and the intravenous route is safer, less traumatic and more effective. Sublingual preparations and suppositories are often not offered to patients but can provide an effective alternative.

Fear of addiction

With the current media messages conveying the dangers of drugs and addiction, coupled with healthcare professionals' irrational concerns with the risk of addiction (Vortherms et al. 1992; Mann 2003), it is no wonder that the general public are reluctant to receive these drugs. The mass media create and convey images of drugs that shape views and have a significant impact on beliefs (Bissel et al. 2001; Morgan and Horne 2005). Nurses may inadvertently make comments such as 'You are better off not taking the stronger ones' or 'We don't want you becoming dependent on them', which only endorse patient concerns. To add to the problem, patients who have been on strong opioids for some time may then experience unpleasant withdrawal symptoms if these are abruptly stopped. This is mistaken for addiction, and the unfortunate patient may then be reluctant to take such drugs again. The issues of addiction, tolerance and dependence are covered in Chapter 4 and that of substance abuse will be covered in more detail in Chapter 7.

Implications of the pain

Patients may worry that when they start to experience pain or their pain increases, this signals the onset of disease progression, for example cancer that has spread. Denying their pain may be part of their coping strategy at this time. Another reason for minimising pain is the fear that discharge home will be delayed: patients may feel that once they are 'pain free', they will be allowed home. It would thus make sense to appear to require little or no medication and deny any discomfort. If you suspect that a patient may be minimising his or her pain, it is essential sensitively to explore the possible reason for this. Some patients feel that their pain should be tolerable because it is '*only* a hernia repair' or 'not as bad as Mrs Black's'. It is important that staff are aware of these perceptions and always assess pain formally.

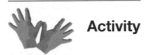 **Activity**

For each of the reasons discussed, identify how you might ensure that patients feel they can be open and honest about their pain. Ask patients about their pain and whether they have been reluctant to report it. Make some notes for each one.

Organisational aspects

Fagerhaugh and Strauss (1977) were the first to look at the organisational setting in which pain management took place and felt that the discrepancy between actual and potential pain relief might be due to the work demands in the clinical area, the lack of accountability surrounding pain management and the complexity of the patient–staff relationship. More recent studies have highlighted similar areas relating to the knowledge of healthcare professionals, poor working relationships and a lack of institutional resources (Brockopp et al. 1998).

It has been acknowledged that legal constraints and institutional policies can unnecessarily limit nurses' ability to manage pain safely and effectively (Jacox et al. 1992; Mann and Carr 2006), but there is little research available that has identified the influence of such policies. Publications advocating putting patients at the centre of healthcare, such as *Creating a Patient-led NHS* (DH 2005), and the introduction of patient group directions (National Prescribing Centre 2004) provide the patient with a stronger voice in practice and may act as a lever to improve pain control. The setting and implementation of minimum standards and the effects of clinical governance may also drive improvements in the way in which we manage pain in the future. A number of initiatives will provide the catalyst for these changes; multidisciplinary working, patient group directions, nurse prescribing, partnerships with patients and users and the increased use of evidence-based practice. Formal documents and policies can improve pain management, a good example of this being the Royal College of Surgeons and the College of Anaesthetists (1990) *Report of the Working Party on Pain after Surgery*. This document resulted in many hospitals forming acute pain teams (see Chapter 4). Let us look now at some of these assumptions in more detail.

Barriers to effective pain management in the clinical area

Work demands

There is no doubt that the pace of work has considerably increased in recent years. Contributing factors such as shortened hospital stay, increased longevity and diminishing resources are implicated. Nurses are busy, doctors are busy, everyone is busy. Lack of time is the most frequently cited barrier to effective pain management (Schafheutle et al. 2001). Carr and Thomas (1997) found that patients' unwillingness to trouble 'busy' staff, even when they were in pain, was a major barrier to obtaining effective pain relief.

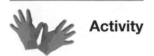 **Activity**

How could you create an environment that oozed a feeling of timelessness in order to encourage patients to stop and ask you for pain relief? This is not easy, but it is worth a try.

In secondary care, creating a relaxing environment is particularly challenging, especially when you are busy. However, in an outpatient environment, for example, gentle instrumental music in the background and the use of plants can provide a feeling of calm. Wherever care takes place, try to maintain eye contact with patients, and always ask open questions regarding their pain. Questions such as 'Tell me about your pain' encourage patients to share their experience with you and suggest to them that you are interested and have time to listen.

Lack of accountability

Although each nurse is held accountable for his or her actions (NMC 2004), the issue about accountability in pain management is not easily resolved. If pain management is not effective, who is to blame? Some may say the doctor did not prescribe the appropriate medication; another might suggest that the nurses did not administer the analgesia regularly enough or question an inadequate prescription. Some hospitals may have an acute pain service, and accountability may be seen to be vested in the 'team' but just how much power and influence do they exert? Similarly, accountability for cancer pain management in the community may be seen to lie with the palliative care or Macmillan team. Nursing staff can be in a key position to be accountable for pain management. They often care for an individual 24 hours a day, and they are the central coordinators for the input of other healthcare professionals, but do we see ourselves as accountable? Nurses also have a key role to play in the development of clinical governance (Moores 1999), but do they always exercise this role to full effect? Improving accountability for the management of pain will be an important part of these endeavours.

Time out

Think about someone you have cared for whose pain was well managed. Who was accountable for their pain management? Now ask some colleagues (including those from other professions) who is accountable for a patient's pain management.

The importance of accountability

Lack of accountability has been implicated as a key factor contributing to ineffective pain management (Lander 1990). You probably found difficulty in identifying one person who held accountability. Some may see the consultant physician as being 'accountable', but does this help when he or she might see the patient only every three days and actually have little up-to-date knowledge of pain management? If the nurse is seen as accountable, but unable to prescribe, this might also present difficulties. There is no clear-cut answer, but nurses have a central role to play, as they are the continuous link between health professionals.

The organisation of nursing care and approaches such as 'primary nursing' and the 'named nurse' were designed to enhance nursing accountability, with advocacy, accountability and individualised care as its central concepts (Pearson 1988). It could be questioned just how successful these initiatives have been, given the slow improvements in pain management especially within acute secondary care.

The delivery of care will continue to evolve, and initiatives such as 'clinical governance' and reaching targets will shape the provision of pain management in the future, increasingly putting pressure on healthcare staff to deliver an improved quality of care. Questions about effectiveness and measurement will act as a catalyst for organisations to evaluate their pain management, and as we have seen in the USA, this may become mandatory in the future. More patient-centred healthcare delivery was the philosophy of *The New National Health Service* (DH 1998) when it was launched, and increasingly healthcare professionals and senior management are being held individually accountable for the delivery of acceptable, humane and knowledgeable practice. Perhaps one way to tackle the slow improvement in pain management would be to link it to the appraisal system.

Institutional policies

The requirement of most hospitals for two nurses to check a controlled drug can increase the length of time over which patients suffer pain, and reducing this to single nurse administration considerably speeds up the delivery of analgesia. Registered nurses dispensing alone currently give far more lethal drugs, for example digoxin, without checking with another practitioner, so why do some hospitals still insist on the outdated practice of two nurses for controlled drugs? Similarly, hospital policy may not allow controlled drugs to be dispensed from the drug trolley, although this could be challenged. The ability to give an oral opioid such as oral morphine syrup from the drug trolley can make a huge difference and at a strength of 10mg in 5ml this very effective analgesic is not classed as a controlled drug, but despite this, it is frequently locked away and double-checked. Clinicians should be encouraged to challenge hospital policies that mitigate against effective pain management. The ability critically to consider the environment one practises in is nothing more than professional, and if policies are found to contribute to ineffective pain management, they should be challenged.

Solutions that avoid tackling organisational policies can be very short-term approaches. Teamworking and discussion with a professional head such as the director of nursing or senior medical consultant can be invaluable. If the problems and possible solutions have been well thought out and evidence of a need for change obtained, it is often extremely satisfying to challenge traditional practice and bring about change that can have far-reaching benefits for patients. Single nurse administration of controlled drugs is a good example (Mann and Redwood 2000).

Changing local policy

All too often, one or two short-acting analgesics are prescribed on a prn basis instead of prescribing regular 'balanced analgesia' to maintain pain relief. A prn prescription tends to ensure that the patient with an ongoing painful condition, which may last for days, experiences a return of pain before asking for further analgesia. This will mean that a higher dose is required to re-establish analgesia, increasing the risk of side effects. By prescribing a range of analgesic drugs, for example an opioid combined with a NSAID and/or paracetamol, matched to the patient's need, titrated to the patient's response and reviewed on a regular basis, far better analgesia can be maintained (McQuay et al. 1997). Patient group directions and nurse prescribing can have a positive impact on the administration and prescribing of effective analgesia. We have found, however, that one of the most effective policies is to agree a hospital-wide protocol for the management of acute pain (which should always respond well to appropriate analgesia). On a practical level, this protocol could include the use of a sticky label attached to each drug chart. An algorithm developed for the administration of intravenous opioids will ensure that following some additional training, nurses can use this route to rapidly establish pain relief, should the situation arise. These strategies will be discussed in more detail in Chapter 4 with examples from practice.

National policies

The modernisation of the NHS coupled with a review of nursing roles have helped to push forward legislation to widen prescribing beyond the medical practitioner.

These changes and influence on local policy are welcome, as they will facilitate a reduction of barriers, which impede the effective and timely administration of analgesics. Three key developments in relation to pain are important; supplementary prescribing, independent nurse prescribing and patient group directions.

Supplementary prescribers are nurses, pharmacists, chiropodists/podiatrists, physiotherapists and radiographers who have undergone specialist training. They can prescribe any NHS medicine provided it is in partnership with an independent prescriber, who establishes the initial diagnosis and starts the treatment. The supplementary prescriber then monitors the patient and prescribes further supplies of medication when necessary. Initially aimed at chronic disease management in primary care, there has been a call for consideration in acute settings if the benefits are to be realised (Fitzpatrick 2004).

In May 2006, qualified nurse independent prescribers (previously known as extended formulary nurse prescribers) were permitted to prescribe any licensed medicine for any medical condition within their competence, including some controlled drugs. A consultation took place in 2007, which will hopefully open the gate to widen prescribing access for nurses (and dentists) to include opioids across several patient groups including postoperative and trauma. A recent national advert for an advanced perioperative practitioner required the applicant to work as an independent prescriber and give oral and parental medicines. The pace of change is fast and a range of healthcare professionals are eligible to take forward these changes in prescribing. Such initiatives are welcome as they can only reduce the barriers imposed in the clinical area by restrictive policies that do little to help practitioners reduce pain and suffering in a timely manner.

National policies in the USA have attempted to bring good pain management practice under review. In 2001 the Joint Commission on Accreditation of Health Care Organizations (JCAHO) incorporated the new standards for pain management, summarised in Chapter 2. The guidelines promoted aggressive treatment of acute pain. Despite the fact that hospital accreditation hinges on the implementation of these guidelines, a study in 2003 appeared to indicate that so far they had had little influence on practice patterns or on improved pain control for patients (Apfelbaum et al. 2003), although this might be slowly changing.

Global policies

It can be difficult to look beyond our local practice and think more widely but there are parallel barriers on a much larger scale, which impede the management of pain for people in certain countries in the world. The Wisconsin Policy Unit in the USA is working globally to reduce the barriers imposed by policies that restrict the effective management of pain (Gilson et al. 2005). Some countries have such stringent policies regarding the import of opioids or narcotics that the medical need for people legitimately experiencing cancer or surgical pain is neglected (Joranson and Ryan 2007). The national 'quota' for importing opioids is linked to each country's drug policy and clearly some governments might prefer not to import these drugs as they cannot be sure they will stay in safe hands. The Wisconsin Policy Unit has produced excellent statistics highlighting the inadequate consumption of opioids in different countries around the world. They also work closely with the World Health Organization to bring expertise from around the world to address issues of pain in cancer.

Conclusion

Effective pain management is challenged by barriers generated by patients, practitioners and their colleagues as well as the organisation in which they practice. Education is probably the most important tool for improving pain management but education alone will not necessarily change practice. There is a need to develop interprofessional education so that healthcare professionals can learn together about pain management. To effect change in practice, there is a need for health professionals to have an understanding of knowledge improvement. The linking together of knowledge about pain and understanding of the mechanisms to effect change can be a critical path to reduce barriers and improve care.

Future changes in healthcare will bring increased pressure for better pain management. The hospital treatment of patients is likely to result in sicker, more dependent individuals being nursed in general wards rather than high dependency units. Early discharge home and increased day case surgery, as well as a larger number of elderly clients, will continue to increase the prevalence of pain in the community. It is essential that practitioners are armed with the most appropriate pain knowledge and can critically consider potential barriers to effective pain management. Although removing barriers may appear to be straightforward once you are aware of them, do not underestimate the challenges ahead.

After a break, try the multiple choice test to self-assess your learning so far. For some of the questions more than one answer will be correct, however, there will be one answer that is so far best supported by the evidence.

Suggested further reading

Institute of Cancer Research and Royal Marsden Hospital (2008) 'Breaking Barriers: Management of Cancer-related Pain', CD-ROM. Information at http://www.ieu.icr.ac.uk.

Middleton C. (2004) Barriers to the provision of effective pain management. *Nursing Times*, **100**(3): 42–5.

Redmond K. (1998) Barriers to the effective management of pain. *International Journal of Palliative Nursing*, 4(6): 276–83.

Van Niekerek L. and Martin F. (2003) The impact of the nurse-physician relationship on barriers encountered by nurses during pain management. *Pain Management Nursing*, 4(1): 3–10.

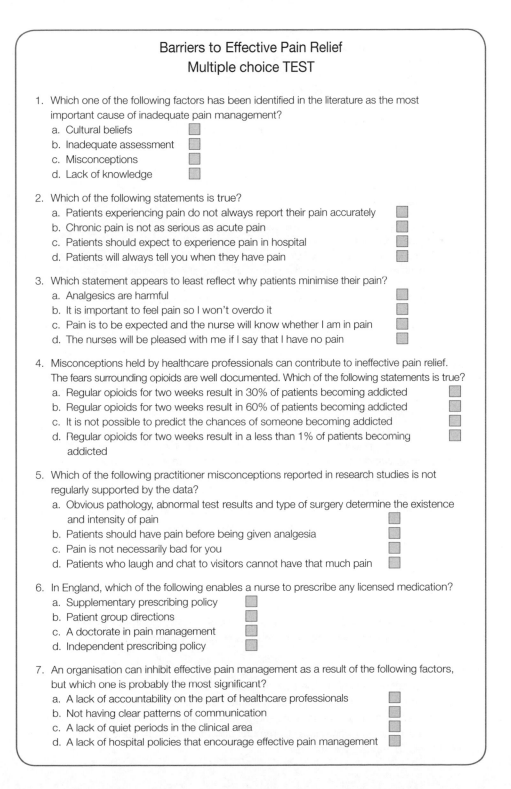

Barriers to Effective Pain Relief
Multiple choice TEST

1. Which one of the following factors has been identified in the literature as the most important cause of inadequate pain management?
   a. Cultural beliefs
   b. Inadequate assessment
   c. Misconceptions
   d. Lack of knowledge

2. Which of the following statements is true?
   a. Patients experiencing pain do not always report their pain accurately
   b. Chronic pain is not as serious as acute pain
   c. Patients should expect to experience pain in hospital
   d. Patients will always tell you when they have pain

3. Which statement appears to least reflect why patients minimise their pain?
   a. Analgesics are harmful
   b. It is important to feel pain so I won't overdo it
   c. Pain is to be expected and the nurse will know whether I am in pain
   d. The nurses will be pleased with me if I say that I have no pain

4. Misconceptions held by healthcare professionals can contribute to ineffective pain relief. The fears surrounding opioids are well documented. Which of the following statements is true?
   a. Regular opioids for two weeks result in 30% of patients becoming addicted
   b. Regular opioids for two weeks result in 60% of patients becoming addicted
   c. It is not possible to predict the chances of someone becoming addicted
   d. Regular opioids for two weeks result in a less than 1% of patients becoming addicted

5. Which of the following practitioner misconceptions reported in research studies is not regularly supported by the data?
   a. Obvious pathology, abnormal test results and type of surgery determine the existence and intensity of pain
   b. Patients should have pain before being given analgesia
   c. Pain is not necessarily bad for you
   d. Patients who laugh and chat to visitors cannot have that much pain

6. In England, which of the following enables a nurse to prescribe any licensed medication?
   a. Supplementary prescribing policy
   b. Patient group directions
   c. A doctorate in pain management
   d. Independent prescribing policy

7. An organisation can inhibit effective pain management as a result of the following factors, but which one is probably the most significant?
   a. A lack of accountability on the part of healthcare professionals
   b. Not having clear patterns of communication
   c. A lack of quiet periods in the clinical area
   d. A lack of hospital policies that encourage effective pain management

8. While in hospital, who do you feel should hold accountability for a patient's pain management?
   a. The patient ☐
   b. The nurse looking after a patient in pain ☐
   c. The medical consultant in charge of the patient's care ☐
   d. The hospital acute pain team ☐

9. Which is probably the most important for improving pain management?
   a. More nursing staff ☐
   b. Education ☐
   c. A wider range of analgesics ☐
   d. Nurse prescribing ☐

10. Which approach to the provision of education in pain management is likely to have the most impact on practice?
   a. Formal lectures in a classroom for nurses of all grades ☐
   b. Lunch-time discussions around a 'patient', involving all professionals ☐
   c. Discussions on the ward rounds ☐
   d. Planned multidisciplinary teaching around a patient case study ☐

Answers

1. d. Lack of knowledge of healthcare professionals seems to be the factor most cited in studies. However, the others are all important factors to consider.
2. a. Patients experiencing pain do not always report their pain accurately; there are numerous reasons why patients might minimise their pain: not wanting to be a bother to the nurses, anxiety about pain delaying their return home, wanting to appear stoic or feeling that it is unacceptable to show that they have pain.
3. d. 'The nurses will be pleased with me if I say I have no pain' does sometimes come up in the literature but the other statements appear quite frequently and should be considered when undertaking a pain assessment. These factors are all powerful inhibitors of effective pain management and can prevent patients expressing their pain. More recent research in the postoperative patient is shedding some light on patients' negative attitudes to analgesia.
4. d. Regular opioids for two weeks results in a less than 1% of patients becoming addicted.
5. c. 'Pain is not necessarily bad for you' is a statement not supported by the evidence; all the other statements have been made by healthcare professionals in a wide range of literature.
6. d. Independent prescribing policy.
7. a. Lack of accountability on the part of healthcare professionals has been reported as one of the main reasons why there is a discrepancy between actual and potential pain relief in the clinical area. The literature suggests that high work demands and rigid hospital policies may also contribute. Communication is also important but accountability would help to improve this as well.

8. b. The nurse looking after a patient in pain is in the best position to take accountability as they spend more time with patients than any other healthcare professional. Patients themselves may feel too ill, too disempowered or just not able to be accountable. Their medical consultant may only see them very briefly over the course of their admission and may not have undertaken any specific education in pain management. The acute pain team may be accountable for general policies and the hospital-wide pain management strategies but it would not be practical or achievable for them to hold accountability for individual patient's pain.

9. b. Education is suggested to be the remedy for the evident lack of knowledge in studies that report on inadequate management of pain. It is unlikely that more nursing staff, nurse prescribing and a wider range of analgesics will have much impact unless those involved have the knowledge to utilise them effectively.

10. d. Planned multidisciplinary teaching around a patient case study offers all those professionals involved in the patient's pain management the chance to participate together. They are more likely to share the difficulties they have encountered, which can be invaluable in promoting effective communication and learning from their experiences. Lunchtime discussions can be a good second best. Formal lectures may not address the difficulties encountered in practice. Ward rounds can be useful, but time and issues of privacy might inhibit fruitful learning.

CHAPTER 4

Managing Acute Pain

Learning outcomes

On completion of this chapter, the student will be able to:

■ Review the pharmacological, psychological, behavioural and physical strategies used in the management of acute pain

■ Critically evaluate current approaches to pain management and their implementation in institutional and non-institutional settings

■ Analyse practices for managing acute pain in his or her own clinical area against current best evidence and identify methods of influencing change

---

Indicative reading

Australian and New Zealand College of Anaesthesia and Faculty of Pain Medicine, (2005) *Acute Pain Management: Scientific Evidence*, 2nd edn. ANZCA, http://www.nhmrc.gov.au/publications/_files/cp104.pdf.

Bandolier, Acute Pain, Oxford Pain Internet Site, http://www.jr2.ox.ac.uk/bandolier/index.html.

Carr D. and Goudas L. (1999) Acute pain. *Lancet*, **353**: 2051–8.

Chapman C., Tuckett R. and Song C. (2007) Pain and stress in a systems perspective: reciprocal neural, endocrine and immune interactions. *Journal of Pain*, 9(2): 122–45.

National Guideline Clearinghouse, Clinical Practice Guidelines for the Management of Postoperative Pain and Assessment and Management of Acute Pain, www.guidelines.gov.

Spearing N., March L., Bellamy N., Bogduk N. and Brooks P. (2005) Management of acute musculoskeletal pain. *APLAR Journal of Rheumatology*, **8**(1): 5–15.

Background

Begin by reading a selection of the literature cited on the previous page. These sources will give you an understanding of some of the current techniques used to manage acute pain and the issues or barriers that contribute to ineffective pain management.

Acute pain commonly occurs in the postoperative period and is associated with injury such as a burn or trauma, infection such as appendicitis or otitis media (earache) and certain diseases and acute conditions such as **myocardial infarction (MI)**. Although following surgery or an injury pain can be predicted, it remains a fact that more than 50% of patients continue to experience severe pain after such events (IASP/European Federation of IASP 2004). Not only does this result in unnecessary suffering, it occurs despite a huge increase in our knowledge of pain, effective treatments for the management of acute pain and now overwhelming evidence that the inadequate treatment of acute pain increases the risk of postoperative complications and may lead to persistent or chronic pain. In fact, it is now suggested that in Western societies, persistent pain following operations and injuries contributes to at least 25% of the burden of chronic pain (Perkins and Kehlet 2000; Bandolier 2002; IASP/European Federation of IASP 2004). In a study of 10 pain clinics to investigate how common chronic pain was in patients after surgery, 23% reported pain, 59% had experienced pain for longer than 24 months, 75% complained that the pain was continuous and 76% reported pain as moderate to severe (Crombie et al. 1998). See Bandolier's (2002) article on chronic pain after surgery for a breakdown of the incidence of chronic pain following a range of common procedures (Table 4.1).

Table 4.1 Incidence of chronic pain after surgery

Procedure	Per cent
Amputation	30–85
Thoracotomy	5–67
Mastectomy	11–57
Cholecystectomy	3–56
Inguinal hernia	0–63
Vasectomy	0–37
Dental surgery	5–13

Although much of the evidence relating to acute pain management comes from the hospital setting, evidence-based principles can be applied to the management of most acutely painful conditions in the community. In this chapter, we will initially explore the concept of acute pain from the patients' viewpoint before considering some of the common interventions. You will be constantly considering the management of acute pain in terms of your own clinical experiences and the findings from research studies in this area. This sets the scene before we explore, in greater detail, the strategies available to manage pain effectively.

Despite the advent of technologies such as patient-controlled analgesia (PCA), continuous epidural analgesia, analgesia pumps, continuous nerve blocks and other implantable devises, the role of the ward or community-based nurse is crucial to the effective delivery of pain care. All too often, however, the most effective strategies are the simpler ones (McQuay et al. 1997). We now have a wealth of guidelines available to us but as we explored in the previous chapter on barriers, it is clear that despite the evidence supporting many of these guidelines, in the main they have failed to decrease patients' pain. It appears that organisations and researchers have ignored the impact of contextual influences on clinicians' decision-making (Bucknall et al. 2001). We will therefore try to suggest practical ways in which some of these problems may be overcome by practice-based clinicians.

The patients' perspective: experiencing acute pain

As previously stated, pain has been defined as 'an unpleasant sensory and emotional experience associated with actual or potential tissue damage, or described in terms of such damage' (IASP 1986 p. 5216). Let us look at how the patient views pain. Before we do this, however, it is important to take a closer look at your ward, unit or community setting.

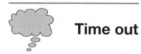 **Time out**

In a day, how many people do you encounter who are experiencing acute pain? Ask family or friends who have had an acute pain experience (surgery or some type of trauma) whether they were offered pain relief quickly. How did they feel? How effective was the treatment they were offered?

Unless they have a rare genetic condition, at one time or another everyone has experienced pain. Interestingly, many people put up with inadequate pain management because of their low expectations concerning pain relief: they may feel that it is an inevitable part of the situation (Carr and Thomas 1997) or they are concerned about taking medication (Older et al. 2007).

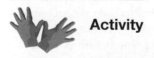 **Activity**

Select two patients and ask them to tell you about their pain. To do this, it is necessary to be fairly unstructured, as you want them to talk as 'openly' as possible and give you plenty of information.

Sample questions are:

- Tell me about your pain.
- What helps your pain?
- What could the nurses do to make your pain better or help you to cope with it more effectively?

Each interview should take 5–10 minutes. Recording (tape or digitally) will save you having to take notes (but always ask the patient's permission first). Otherwise, write down as much as you can. Include your observations of the patient (facial expression, body language and so on).

Although acute pain is usually associated with a specific event, we sometimes consider only trauma and surgical intervention to be the causes of acute pain, but what about other procedures that patients frequently undergo such as dressing changes, catheter insertion, dental treatment, venepuncture, drain removal, suturing and stitch removal? In *Giving Comfort and Inflicting Pain*, Madjar (1998) writes vividly about her interviews with burn patients and patients receiving chemotherapy. The book narrates the lived experience of pain inflicted in the context of prescribed medical treatment. It explores pain from the perspective of the patients who endured it and the nurses whose actions contributed.

 Time out

Reflect on the findings from your interviews. What are the implications for your practice? Why treat acute pain?

While it is unethical to allow patients to suffer, it is also extremely detrimental to their recovery. If postoperative pain is acute and uncontrolled, the patient is unlikely to move, preferring to lie as still as possible to avoid inducing further pain. Particularly when combined with the stress response to trauma or surgery, this can have several unwanted side effects, some of which are potentially very serious:

- Respiratory function, for example, may be compromised, and coughing and deep breathing avoided, predisposing to chest infection or even lung collapse (atelectasis).
- Pain is linked to tachycardia and hypertension, increasing the likelihood of MI in susceptible patients who have a history of heart disease.
- Pain and stress increase platelet adhesion, which may increase the risk of developing DVT and pulmonary embolism (PE).
- The stress response also increases the metabolic rate, contributing to immunosuppression and an increased risk of infection.

- Gastrointestinal function can become compromised, increasing the risk of ileus (reduced gut motility).
- Pain can cause significant sleep disturbances, which can lead to fatigue and limit daytime energy, increasing the incidence and severity of depression and mood disturbances.
- Inactivity can rapidly lead to deconditioning, gait disturbances and, in the elderly, an increased risk of injuries from falls.
- Uncontrolled pain is a contributing factor to postoperative nausea and vomiting. This can then slow recovery through dehydration, wound dehiscence and haemorrhage.
- The societal consequences of pain include the increased financial and caring burdens placed on families and friends as well as the expensive increased utilisation of healthcare services.

All these consequences of pain are not only potentially dangerous for the individual, they also diminish the quality of life and slow recovery. They are also costly for the hospitals treating complications and the community-based services providing after-care. However, the implications for hospitals and community trusts are not only the financial impact, as we move to more target-driven healthcare, but also poor pain management may lead to adverse outcome measures reflected in league tables. In the USA, inadequate pain management can now lead to the loss of accreditation if a hospital fails to comply with set minimum standards. There have also been legal precedents in the USA involving the undertreatment of patients in pain. For example, in one case in California, the family of a man who died in pain successfully sued his doctor. This doctor had been reluctant to prescribe opioids. As a result of this case, it became law that all doctors in the state of California have to undertake at least 12 hours of pain education (Charatan 2001).

In the past, we have underestimated the damage that pain may cause. We now know that the consequences of immobilisation-induced organ dysfunction, impaired pulmonary function, **hypoxemia**, myocardial **ischemia** and so on cannot be overemphasised. As healthcare comes under increasing scrutiny to deliver safe and effective care, with positive outcomes and value for money, we hope that the consequences of poor pain control will achieve the higher priority they deserve.

Acute pain services

The concept of the 'acute pain service' (APS) originated in the USA, led by an anaesthetist called Brian Ready in Seattle. It was to provide a template for development of services in the UK (Ready et al. 1988). A report from the Royal College of Surgeons and College of Anaesthetists (1990) concluded that the traditional methods of managing pain after surgery, for example opioid analgesia given intramuscularly, were inadequate and recommended that an APS be introduced into all major hospitals performing surgery in the UK. By 1995, 57% of hospitals had an acute pain team (Windsor et al. 1996), and by 2004, well over a decade after the recommendation, this had finally risen to 89.4% (Nagi 2004).

The acute pain service or team usually comprises an anaesthetist, an acute pain clinical nurse specialist and sometimes a pharmacist or other clinician such as a physiotherapist. Some teams may also be able to call on the services of a clinical psychologist, although this is probably quite rare. The team is responsible for the day-to-day management of pain after surgery and trauma, and for ensuring that adequate monitoring is available for the pain-relieving technique chosen, for example epidural analgesia or PCA. Education features prominently, and many run in-service training on analgesic techniques as well as on pain-related topics. In many hospital wards, nurses now routinely care for patients receiving epidural analgesia, whereas a few years ago, these patients would have been nursed in an intensive care or high dependency unit. Some teams also undertake research related to pain, and it is standard practice for them all to audit the service continuously in order to evaluate the effectiveness of any new initiatives.

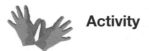

Time out

Think about how the role of the ward nurse in managing pain has changed over the past 10 years. Can you foresee any negative aspects?

The role of the ward nurse is critical to the success of the endeavours of the acute pain team, and it has been suggested that hospital nurses need further education to enable them to broaden their role in pain management (Bucknall et al. 2001). There was a concern that the role of ward nurses might be eroded as they see 'experts' taking responsibility for pain management (Notcutt 1997). It is essential, therefore, that nurses are empowered to take responsibility for pain management and to adopt an active role in assessing pain and evaluating the effectiveness of interventions. Very few acute pain services can offer 24-hour cover and the quality of pain management should be consistent whether there is more expert backup or not.

Activity

If ward nurses are to be 'empowered', how might this be done? If you are based in secondary care, what is the role of the APS in your hospital? Does the team see all patients with PCA and epidurals, or do the ward nurses only call the team if there are problems?

In primary care, do you have access to a clinician with a special interest and extended knowledge about pain and its management?

Case history

You are looking after a 68-year-old gentleman called Mr Henderson who you consider to be in a great deal of pain following an abdominal operation. He doesn't want to cause a fuss and you feel that his verbal report of pain control as being 'OK' doesn't give the true picture. Trying to assess his pain intensity using a numerical scale or verbal rating proves frustrating as he just states he is in pain but he'll be all right and is reluctant to give you a particular rating. As soon as you try to get him to move or he gives a little cough, his body language and facial grimacing indicate that he is extremely uncomfortable and it is obvious he is unable to mobilise effectively. You look at his medication chart and although he has been administered regular paracetamol and the prescribed dose of 10mg oral morphine (prn – as required) has been given on five occasions over 24 hours, you feel his analgesia is inadequate. It is the weekend, no one from the pain team is available, and you waste a considerable amount of time trying to locate a doctor but most of them are busy on another ward or in theatre seeing to an emergency. When you approach a senior nurse who is also very busy, she asks the patient if he is all right and, as you expect, he smiles and states he's fine. Meanwhile, more time elapses and his pain appears to get worse. Frustratingly, his oral morphine has been prescribed as a single dose (rather than a dose range) of 10mg 4-hourly prn and he was last given this only an hour ago. You feel angry and powerless to resolve this situation quickly.

Possible solution:
In the short term, you are only left with reassurance and non-pharmacological therapies such as comfort strategies while you wait for a doctor to change the prescription. Non-pharmacological therapies have an important place; however, if postoperative pain is severe, their role can be somewhat limited. Although a new protocol would take time to devise, agree and implement, a possible long-term solution to this common problem could be the introduction of a pre-printed sticky label to enable a wider range of pharmacological strategies to be used in combination and at dosages that can be adjusted to individual need.

An example of a sticky label currently used in a district general hospital for the management of all acute and trauma pain is given in Figure 4.1. This begins with paracetamol to which ibuprofen may be added if not contraindicated. It also includes both intravenous and oral morphine, which may then be administered if a combination of full dose, regular paracetamol and ibuprofen fail to control pain. Combining non-opioids with opioids produces a synergistic effect and has the potential to enable reduced doses of opioids to be given, thereby reducing side effects (Kehlet 1997). It also enables pain to be rapidly brought under control, removing the potential for delays that were such a common feature and were highlighted in this case history.

ADULTS ONLY
Signature Date Bleep No.   Pharmacy V3
MORPHINE I.V I.V assesed staff only 1mg I.V prn – max 10mg Use APS protocol for guidance on dose and time

PARACETAMOL

Route:	Dose:	Frequency:
P.O/P.R	1mg	QDS

IBUPROFEN
Delete if NSAID contraindicated

Route:	Dose:	Frequency:
P.O/S.L	400mg	TDS

ORAL MORPHINE
10mg/5ml
Omit during epidural or PCA

Age guide:	Dose:	Frequency:
16–70 yrs	10–30mgs	3–6 hrly
>70 yrs	5–10mgs	4–6 hrly

ONDANSETRON

Route:	Dose:	Frequency:
I.V/P/O	4mg	8 hrly

MAGNESIUM HYDROXIDE
(Laxative)
Delete in bowel or abdominal
surgery patients

Route:	Dose:	Frequency:
P.O	20–40ml	nocte

Figure 4.1 An example of a sticky label covering a range of analgesia to treat acute pain

Source: By kind permission of Poole Hospital NHS Trust

The label also includes strategies to counteract the inevitable side effects experienced by many individuals when opioids are administered. You will notice that weak opioids, such as codeine, have been excluded. This is because evidence suggests that paracetamol and ibuprofen are both more effective than any of the weak opioids alone (Bandolier 2005). This is covered later in the chapter. Although on this occasion, the patient is able to take oral medications, if analgesia needs to be re-established rapidly in a patient with intravenous access, it can be very useful for nurses to be able to immediately titrate intravenous morphine. Figure 4.2 provides an example of an algorithm to assist nursing staff in the safe and effective administration of intravenous opioids. Being able to rapidly move up to stronger analgesia when needed can lead to a dramatic improvement in patients' experience of pain control (Layzell 2005). A criticism of the label is that to get the policy agreed, the analgesia was printed as prn only. We know from research that prn does not optimise pain control unless the return of pain is pre-empted and further analgesia given before previous doses wear off. Pain control is achieved much more effectively by 'round-the-clock', regular dosages.

ALGORITHIM FOR ADMINISTRATION OF INTRAVENOUS OPIOIDS DILUTED IN 10mls NORMAL SALINE

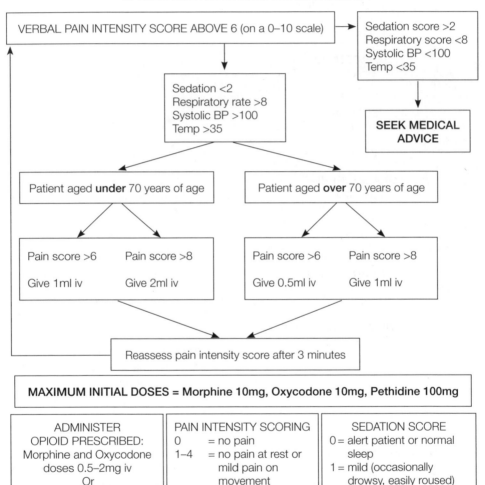

Figure 4.2 Algorithm for administration of intravenous opioids

Source: By kind permission of Poole Hospital NHS Trust

Case history

Returning to Mr Henderson, in the short term, all you can do is keep trying to locate a doctor so you can get his prescription altered to increase the opioid dosage, shorten the time between doses (1–2-hourly should be quite safe if patients are assessed appropriately), maybe consider regular titrated opioid analgesia for 24 hours or so and also consider adding in a NSAID if these drugs are well tolerated. In a modern hospital in the twenty-first century, no patient should be left in pain because their analgesia prescription is inadequate.

There is no doubt that the introduction of new pain technologies and encouraging different ways of using existing drugs has done much to improve the quality of pain relief for most patients. The future may see the natural development of acute pain teams into 'perioperative care' teams, where nutrition, fluid balance, the prevention of DVT and mobilisation complement their role in the provision of analgesia. This is already happening in Denmark, and there is much discussion on the **multimodal** approach to improve recovery, prevent the unwanted side effects of surgery and speed up discharge (Kehlet and Holt 2001).

All too often, healthcare professionals do not explore patients' views on their pain management but focus instead on pharmacological interventions. Strategies such as relaxation, distraction, information-giving, comfort (positioning) and being with the patient can all contribute to the reduction of pain or help patients to 'cope' with their pain more effectively. These strategies can have the additional benefit of reducing the dosages of analgesia and enhancing their effect. You may have found that the patients to whom you have spoken mentioned non-pharmacological strategies that helped them control their pain; we will cover some of these strategies later on in the chapter.

 Time out

Think about the interventions commonly used to manage acute pain in your area. Make a list of these to review later.

In the next section, we will consider the various types of drug used in the pharmacological management of acute pain and consider some of the current methods of administration, such as PCA, continuous epidural and nerve blocks as well as further strategies to maximise analgesic administration such as multimodal therapy. It is important to complement pharmacological interventions with non-pharmacological approaches and strategies to combine therapies will be explored later in the chapter.

Pharmacological approaches to pain management

Analgesics are some of the most common 'over-the-counter' (OTC) drugs, but knowledge is required to optimise their effectiveness. It is essential to teach patients how drugs work, their possible side effects and how to avoid these. In the community where patients self-administer their analgesics, it is also important to ascertain the barriers to their use. Many a bathroom cabinet can be found crammed full of unused prescribed analgesics that were never taken properly or effectively. Although doctors within the hospital setting generally prescribe analgesics, the administration of analgesia to the patient is viewed as primarily a nursing role. It is necessary, therefore, that nurses are knowledgeable in pharmacology and are able to apply this knowledge critically to their practice.

Knowledge of analgesia in terms of dose, effectiveness, side effects and how drugs can be combined to give balanced or multimodal analgesia is the basis of good pain relief. There is no great myth or complexity to this – just clear understanding and confidence. Nurses also need to educate patients not only on the side effects of analgesia, but also the rationale for their use. Many patients (and healthcare professionals) are reluctant to take analgesia, but a clear understanding of why it is important to be comfortable will encourage patients to accept pain relief and report its inadequacies.

Commonly used analgesics

To indicate visually the various forms in which these drugs are available, we have used the following symbols:

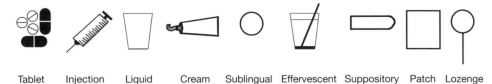

| Tablet | Injection | Liquid | Cream | Sublingual preparation | Effervescent solution | Suppository | Patch | Lozenge |

Analgesics for mild to moderate pain

Paracetamol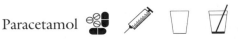

Most of us have used this drug at some time. It is useful for mild-to-moderate pain and can be used in combination with other drugs for pain that fails to respond adequately as it can considerably increase the effectiveness of other analgesics. For example, with codeine 60mg, you need to give the drug to approximately 17 patients for one patient to achieve a 50% reduction of their pain score (the efficacy of analgesics being expressed as the number needed to treat (NNT) – the lower the number, the better). If 1g paracetamol is given with 60mg codeine, the NNT is reduced to around 3. See McQuay et al. (1997) for further information on NNTs and analgesia.

Paracetamol is also useful for lowering the temperature. It is thought to work by predominantly inhibiting the body's synthesis of prostaglandin in the central nervous system.

Paracetamol is sometimes regarded as a NSAID, but this is not the case, as it has no effect on inflammation (Soberman and Christmas 2003).

Paracetamol does not appear to have a strong effect at the peripheral level, therefore does not produce gastric irritation and does not affect platelet function. Paracetamol is useful for non-inflammatory pain such as a headache or muscle ache but is not particularly good on its own for severe pain. It can be highly toxic if taken as an overdose, and as it has a **ceiling effect**, there is no point in exceeding the recommended dose. For persistent pain, it is usually best taken on a regular basis to maintain a steady state concentration in the blood. It is now available in an intravenous form, which is particularly useful for postoperative patients who cannot take oral medications in the immediate postoperative period.

Non steroidal anti-inflammatory drugs (NSAIDS)

Non-steroidal anti-inflammatory drugs (NSAIDs) form a large group of drugs that reduce inflammation and come in a wide range of formats. Most of them produce some analgesia after just one dose, but they are usually best given regularly to reduce any swelling, muscle tenderness or joint stiffness. They are particularly useful following sports injury, for arthritis and menstrual cramping. Like paracetamol, these drugs affect the body's synthesis of prostaglandin, but the NSAIDs do this mostly at the site of tissue damage. They are very good for mild-to-moderate pain and will sometimes be useful for even quite severe pain. They are also of benefit when given with opioid analgesics, providing additional analgesia that can reduce the need to escalate to larger doses. There is also a ceiling effect for NSAIDs, so exceeding the recommended dose will not achieve better analgesia and could greatly increase the risk of potentially dangerous side effects. In some studies, NSAIDs provided pain relief equivalent to or even better than 10mg intramuscular morphine (McQuay and Moore 1998).

There is a vast range of these drugs, which can be given in a variety of ways. If a patient taking a NSAID obtains only disappointing relief of their pain, it is sometimes worthwhile changing to another NSAID from a different chemical class. Table 4.2 lists some popular NSAIDs divided into their chemically related groups.

Two types of NSAID must, however, *never* be given together, as this may result in serious side effects.

Table 4.2 Popular NSAIDs divided into their chemically related groups

Group 1	Group 2	Group 3	Group 4	Group 5
Ibuprofen	Diclofenac	Indomethacin	Piroxicam	Mefenamic acid
Naproxen	Ketorolac			

Aspirin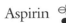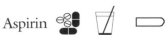

The oldest NSAID and probably the most familiar is aspirin. Like all NSAIDs, aspirin is particularly useful for providing analgesia while reducing both temperature and inflammation. Its effect on inhibiting platelet aggregation is such that it is given as a **prophylactic** to reduce the risk of clot formation in vascular disease. Unfortunately, it is very irritant to the stomach, and can cause a severe asthmatic attack in about 5–10% of patients who have developed adult-onset asthma. However, if an asthmatic patient has used aspirin in the past with no ill effect, it is safe to use it again. It is also not recommended for children because of the risk of **Reye's syndrome**, an acute, life-threatening illness.

Ibuprofen

Ibuprofen is another commonly used NSAID and like aspirin is available over the counter in most countries, because at a low dose, it probably has the best side effect profile. While NSAIDs such as ibuprofen relieve pain and inflammation much like aspirin does, they do not affect blood clotting in the same way. In fact, some research indicates that taking ibuprofen regularly seems to inhibit aspirin's ability to prevent a first heart attack (Kurth et al. 2003). Common to all NSAIDs, some asthmatics will not be able to tolerate ibuprofen because it brings on wheezing. Although a potentially serious side effect, many asthmatics do appear to be able to tolerate ibuprofen, with a study in the US finding the prevalence of ibuprofen-sensitive asthma in children to be low at around 2–4% (Debley et al. 2005).

Although NSAIDs are usually very effective, especially following injury or surgery, they can have some particularly serious side effects that limit their use – especially in the elderly or those with gastric, cardiac or renal problems. Many of these side effects are seen with long-term use, so the administration of NSAIDs for only a few days appears to be relatively safe. Some NSAIDs are also available as topical preparations, and these may be well worth a trial: topical NSAIDs are not associated with the gastrointestinal adverse effects that are seen with the same drugs taken orally (Evans et al. 1995).

COX-2 specific NSAIDs

New types of NSAID described as COX-2 specific are currently available, which, because of their selective action, are considered safer for patients with a history of gastric ulceration. However, more recent concerns have been raised about their use in patients with cardiovascular disease and certain skin disorders. Up-to-date advice should be obtained, since several of these medications have been withdrawn in the past few years (see Medicines and Healthcare Products Regulatory Agency 2007 or US Food and Drug Administration 2007).

For postoperative patients, it has been argued that the risks associated with the side effects of NSAIDs are sometimes overemphasised, as they will only be required for a limited time. Provided that they are prescribed with care, and nurses are aware of what to look for in patients who may be adversely affected by the drugs, the majority of patients can benefit from the pain-relieving properties of NSAIDs. As always, good assessment and monitoring are the key to safe administration in at-risk groups.

Opioids and their use

Opioids come in a range of effectiveness from weak to strong. In their strongest form, they can be used as a first-line drug for pain of such severity that milder drugs are not expected to provide adequate relief. This is particularly the case following any painful surgery or trauma. Whether they are given in their strongest or their weakest form, they can also be combined with paracetamol, aspirin or another NSAID as multimodal therapy, so can be useful when one drug alone fails to provide adequate analgesia. Opioids are best used for dull pain, that is, pain that travels to the spinal cord via the C fibres (see Chapter 1). Opioids act by binding to opioid receptors principally distributed throughout the central nervous system, thereby modulating the transmission of pain impulses. Opioids are not very effective for sharp incident pain, that is, pain transmitted via the A delta fibres. It is also true that only some chronic pain syndromes respond well to opioids. As recent research has indicated, it is not necessarily because the pain is entirely opioid resistant, but more that intolerably high doses, leading to adverse side effects, are needed before any reduction in pain is evident. However, for severe pain following trauma or an operation, for an acutely painful medical condition, or for patients with cancer pain, strong opioids can provide powerful pain relief that is hard to equal with any other analgesia other than nerve block.

To simplify matters, we will just concentrate on the most commonly used opioids, starting with the weaker drugs: codeine and dihydrocodeine.

The weaker opioids

Codeine

This drug comes from the opium poppy and was the mainstay of analgesia for many years. Recently, however, its efficacy versus side effect profile has brought it and other weak opioids under increasing scrutiny (McQuay and Moore 1998) and there is now debate as to whether drugs such as codeine really have a place (Sachs 2005). It is biotransformed in the body to morphine but is much less potent. Research indicates that between 7–10%, and maybe more, of the population are unable to bioconvert codeine and are therefore exposed to the side effects without obtaining any analgesic benefit (Eckhard et al. 1998).

It is usually given in doses of 30–60mg; frequently as a combined preparation with paracetamol. Although doses above 90mg may still be effective in certain individuals, the side effects usually preclude amounts larger than this. Codeine can cause severe constipation and, when used for the first time, usually leaves people feeling drowsy and light-headed. The dose that can be bought over the counter in combined analgesic preparations is very small – no more than 8mg and probably of little additional benefit.

Dihydrocodeine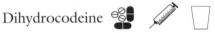

This is a derivative of codeine and is slightly more potent. Although the side effects are the same as for codeine, it may cause more confusion and disorientation, especially in children and the elderly. Again, like codeine, a percentage of the population will be poor metabilisers of this drug.

Tramadol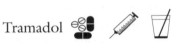

Tramadol is a centrally acting, synthetic analgesic sometime referred to as a weak opioid because it binds very weakly to the mu-opioid receptors. However, it also inhibits the reuptake of other neurotransmitters associated with modulating the pain experience. Like all the opioids, it can cause constipation, nausea and somnolence but it is now available in longer acting formulations such as twice-daily or even a once-daily preparation, with suggestions that in these formats, the incidence and severity of adverse events may be reduced (Mongin 2007). Unlike simple analgesia, tramadol has also been found to be useful for neuropathic pain (Hollingshead et al. 2006).

The following case history illustrates how even a small change in a drug regime can improve a patient's pain control.

Case history

You have an elderly patient called Mr George on your ward who has been taking a co-preparation prescribed by his doctor of paracetamol 500mg with codeine 8mg (co-codamol) one or two tables for many years to control pain from an arthritic hip. He cannot tolerate NSAIDs on a regular basis as he has a history of peptic ulcer disease and has had two MIs in the past. He has now been admitted to hospital for investigations of an unrelated condition but has found that his increased immobility and the anxiety of being in hospital are making his hip pain more difficult to control. What would you suggest?

Possible solution:
As the co-codamol that Mr George takes regularly contains only a very low dose of a weak opioid, he might benefit from taking a full dose of paracetamol 1gm (two tablets) with a variable dose of oral morphine syrup, which can be carefully titrated to optimise benefit or until side effects become unacceptable. It is likely that, given his advanced years, a low dose of 5–10mg oral morphine will give him increased benefit with minimal side effects, as he is already used to taking an opioid, albeit at a non-therapeutic dose. If this still fails to control Mr George's pain adequately, provided he is not experiencing side effects, the morphine can be gradually increased. However, should morphine cause side effects, it is often worth switching to a low dose of a different opioid such as oxycontin in either immediate-release or slow-release format. Although there appears to be sparse published evidence, in our clinical practice, this drug appears to be gentler on the older patient. You may find that the stronger analgesia provides such superior pain relief that Mr George is discharged on this combination and as a result is able to increase his mobility once he has recovered from his hospital admission. As should happen with all patients prescribed opioids, Mr George will need to be given advice, both oral and written, as well as prescribed an aperient, should constipation prove problematic. Not all patients will find they need a laxative if advice on a change to a high-fibre diet with plenty of fluids is followed.

Stronger opioids

Morphine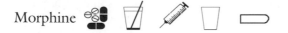

Morphine, like codeine, has its origins in the opium poppy. Its powerful effects have been known for a very long time: in fact there is evidence that these poppies have been cultivated since the third century BC.

Although by no means an ideal drug, or one that will work for all types of pain, morphine still remains the 'gold standard' by which all other pain-relieving drugs are judged. In the authors' experience, it is often underused for moderate-to-severe acute pain. It is frequently observed that a dose of oral morphine, titrated to the patient's response, will produce rapid and adequate analgesia with fewer side effects than a large dose of a weaker opioid. We have also found that oral morphine syrup is particularly useful for children, who should never be subjected to intramuscular analgesia, and who appear to be more at risk of inadequate prescribing than adults. Surprisingly few studies have been conducted on the use of oral morphine syrup, and it could be that a resistance to the extensive use of this preparation is the result of myth and misconception rather than of well-conducted trials that form the basis of evidence-based practice. The drug has no patent on it and is cheap to produce, so doesn't benefit from expensive marketing campaigns.

Diamorphine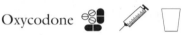

Although this drug is converted in the body to morphine, it is said to have a faster onset of action with a shorter duration of effect. It can be dissolved in a very small quantity of water or saline, which is beneficial for patients needing a continuous subcutaneous infusion. For example, 60mg diamorphine in 10ml normal saline attached to a small portable infusion pump can be delivered over 24 hours.

The drug suffers from an image problem, especially in the USA, where it is not available. It is quite simply heroin, its name alone seeming to arouse horror, especially among the general public. In fact, it can provide superb pain relief, being slightly more potent than morphine and producing slightly more of a euphoric effect. In addition, the physical characteristics that make it soluble in water and fat make it very useful as an epidural, spinal or even intranasal analgesic. Its action when administered into the cerebrospinal fluid or epidural space is more predictable than the action of a water-soluble opioid such as morphine.

Oxycodone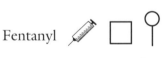

Oxycodone is a strong opioid that acts at the mu- and kappa-opioid receptors and is a little more potent than morphine. It can be useful for patients who are experiencing unacceptable side effects with morphine. Although the side effect profile is similar to morphine, in our experience, changing a patient to oxycodone can reduce itching, sedation, confusion and nausea in some patients and there is now some preliminary literature to support this (Gallego et al. 2007). The drug comes in several formulations including a combined immediate- and extended-release biphasic preparation, which starts to act rapidly but can extend analgesia to 12 hours. Oxycodone has also proved useful in managing neuropathic pain (Riley et al. 2008S).

Fentanyl

Fentanyl is a short-acting opioid 80 times more powerful than morphine. It is used extensively in operating theatres and intensive care units but is now available in a wider range of formats, which has greatly extended its therapeutic application. For example, it is used in a patch for chronic pain particularly in palliative care, and in a lollipop format for rapid transmucosal absorption, which is useful for breakthrough or incident pain, although it is only currently licensed in the UK for patients with malignant disease. It features widely as the opioid component of combined opioid/ local anaesthetic continuous epidurals and has also been used in PCA as an alternative to morphine. Again, its side effect profile is similar to other opioids but it appears to cause less constipation, nausea and vomiting in patch format. Fentanyl does not lead to the accumulation of potentially toxic metabolites and can therefore be used 'with caution' in patients with renal problems.

Methadone

In many industrialised countries, methadone is used extensively to treat drug addiction and is rarely used to control acute pain. It is a powerful analgesic, about as potent as morphine, but it lasts longer and can, when used regularly, accumulate, causing problems. It is, however, useful when morphine is not providing adequate analgesia or it can be used as part of opioid rotation, whereby opioids are switched periodically to achieve a better balance between analgesia and side effects (Fallon 1997). Methadone also binds to the NMDA receptor which is implicated in the development of wind-up and central sensitisation that we touched on in Chapter 1. This could revive the use of methadone particularly for those deemed at risk of developing chronic pain syndrome.

Pethidine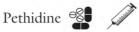

Pethidine is only about one-tenth as potent as morphine, with poor bioavailability when given by mouth. It also has a very short duration of action: somewhere between one and three hours. A serious problem is its metabolite norpethidine, which can accumulate when large doses of the drug are given or it is used for longer than a few days. Norpethidine is toxic and may cause convulsions. These days, given the range of alternative opioids available, there is little advantage to pethidine.

The old idea that pethidine was better than other opioids as a treatment for colicky pain, especially biliary and renal colic, is now discounted (Nagle and McQuay 1990; McQuay 1999). A further note of caution is that this drug can be dangerous if given to a patient taking a monoamine oxidase inhibitor; the combination has been known to send patients spiralling into a hypertensive crisis. Certainly in clinical practice, when the drug was used more extensively, we saw a problem with pethidine addiction, which we didn't see with more longer acting opioids. Such is the disenchantment with this drug that several countries, particularly Australia, have severely curtailed its use or banned it altogether (Davis 2004; Kaye et al. 2005).

Nalbuphine

Nalbuphine (Nubain) is different as it is an antagonist at one opioid receptor, the mu, but acts as an agonist at the kappa receptor. The continued agonist–antagonist action means that there is a ceiling effect for both analgesia and side effects. The drug does not come under the same administration and storage controls as the opioids previously mentioned. Because of these factors, it was widely used by ambulance staff for patients on their way to A&E departments before clinicians became more familiar and comfortable using morphine. It is only available for parenteral administration, which limits its use elsewhere, and more recently, it was discovered that it produces greater analgesia in females than males. In fact, it may increase pain in males, a further reason for it to fall out of favour (Gear et al. 2008).

Buprenorphine ○ ☐

Buprenorphine (Temgesic) is a partial agonist and is about 50 times more potent than morphine. The fact that it is long lasting (acting for about 8–10 hours) and comes as a sublingual preparation and now in a patch format widens its therapeutic application. It is supposed to cause less physical dependence and constipation. It appears to be one of the safer opioids for patients with renal problems when morphine may not be the opioid of choice (Filitz et al. 2005). From a patient's point of view, they seem to either love or hate this drug – those who hate it complaining of excessive nausea and light-headedness. The advent of patch technology may now have overcome some of these problems, because of the slower onset of action and the very low starting doses that can now be initiated.

Naloxone

Naloxone (Narcan) has no other action than to reverse the effects of opioids. It is, therefore, used to reverse an opioid overdose. Its administration often needs to be repeated as it has a short duration of action and opioid action will return within about half an hour. It will not necessarily reverse a partial agonist such as buprenorphine. Used in small doses, that is, 0.2mg, it is also excellent for reversing opioid-induced urinary retention; it has often removed the need to catheterise a patient, much to their relief. In the same small dose, it can be used to treat an opioid-induced itch that does not respond to a dose of antihistamine. If you wish, return briefly to Chapter 1 to refresh your memory on the physiology of opioid action.

For a useful and provocative discourse on opioids, see McQuay (1999). Although this article focuses primarily on chronic and cancer pain, many of the principles apply also to acute pain.

Time out

Think of a patient who has been taking an opioid other than morphine. Was there any reason indicated for why they were taking that particular drug? If you get the chance, ask the prescribing doctor why he or she chose it. Unfortunately, you may still find that prescribing habit and tradition rather than the available evidence have influenced the choice of drug.

Before we leave these brief descriptions of common analgesics, it may be useful to add a little on the way drugs that are not regarded as traditional analgesics are being included in some perioperative pain control regimes. Although not yet standard practice, there have been interesting reports of improving pain control by adding in drugs such as gabapentin and ketamine. Gabapentin is an anticonvulsant that is being increasingly used to treat neuropathic pain and ketamine is an anaesthetic drug that acts as an antagonist at the NMDA receptor. Both these drugs are showing promise as part of a multimodal regime to improve pain control, reduce the doses of opioid required and therefore their side effects and maybe even reduce the risk of chronic post-surgical pain. For more information on these two interesting drugs, see Bell et al. (2006) and Kong and Irwin (2007).

Addiction, tolerance and dependence

We touched on the subject of addiction in Chapter 3 when discussing barriers. Because myths continue to inhibit effective pain control, it is appropriate to expand a little on common concerns at this point.

The literature reveals that not only patients and their carers but also healthcare professionals have serious misgivings regarding the use of opioids in clinical practice, usually based on a lack of knowledge regarding the mechanisms that come into play when opioids are used regularly. When many of our more senior staff were training, Ferrell et al. (1992) reviewed 14 nursing textbooks and discovered that most of them gave inaccurate definitions of addiction, tolerance and dependence. This confusion needs to be clarified.

Addiction

Addiction refers to a psychological dependence characterised by an overwhelming craving for a drug. The addicted individual becomes completely preoccupied with obtaining the drug, but not for its pain-relieving properties. He or she becomes a compulsive drug user who displays loss of control and persistent use despite harm from the drug (Ferrell et al. 1992). The risk of addiction following the use of opioids for pain relief is very small, but many healthcare professionals are still ignorant of this fact and harbour unnecessary and sometimes irrational fears about addiction, thinking that everyone who needs to take opioids for more than a very short time will be at risk.

For example, in a 1990 survey of 2,459 nurses, over 20% believed that addiction occurred in more than 25% of patients receiving opioids for pain (McCaffery et al. 1990). In 2002, these problems persisted, with little change in the data (McCaffery and Robinson 2002). Another survey in 1992 of 243 US physicians found that 20% believed addiction to be a serious problem in patients with cancer pain (Elliott and Elliott 1992) and again, this hadn't changed by 2000 (Score and Attribute 2000). Even when a patient has a prior history of substance abuse, his or her risk of becoming addicted to opioids used for pain relief is very small, probably less than 1% (Ferrell et al. 1992). In a retrospective review of 24,000 patients without a previous history of substance abuse who received opioids for pain relief, approximately 0.3% became addicted. Most of our fears surrounding addiction in patients taking opioids for pain relief are thus completely unfounded. Nevertheless, the mixed messages we all receive as governments and law enforcement agencies try to curb drug use, often via powerful messages in the media, seem to ensure that many patients and professionals will resist the use of opioids for fear of risking addiction.

Tolerance

Patients sometimes appear to get used to a drug and may develop a need for larger doses of opioids in order to control pain. This does not mean, however, that opioid tolerance is going to become a major problem. In fact, tolerance to some opioid side effects, such as sedation and respiratory depression, occurs normally during administration and enables larger doses of the drug to be administered in order to achieve improved analgesia. Most studies show that, with cancer pain, an increase in analgesia requirement is most probably related to disease progression and increased pain rather than a higher tolerance to the drugs (Tywcross 1999; Jage 2005).

Dependence

Physical dependence describes the characteristics of withdrawal symptoms displayed by patients if their opioid dose is significantly reduced or abruptly stopped. These symptoms are not necessarily just a feature of long-term opioid use: it is quite possible for patients to display withdrawal symptoms following intensive opioid administration over a relatively short period of time (Wall and Melzack 1994). Signs of physical withdrawal, which can be very unpleasant for the patient, are easily overcome as long as patients do not discontinue their treatment abruptly. Just as one would treat patients who have received another class of drug that mimics substances produced naturally by the body – steroids – it is important to ensure that patients transfer to a tapering dose schedule when opioid dose reduction is indicated.

The best measures to minimise these consequences depend upon an accurate assessment of pain with the patient and then regular monitoring of the efficacy of pain-relieving therapy. This will help healthcare professionals to select appropriate strategies to manage the pain effectively, ensuring that the dose of drug is appropriate when pain is severe but tapered off once the pain starts to resolve. Working with other healthcare professionals and helping them to overcome any misconceptions they may have must also be part of the process, in order to ensure effective pain relief. The British Pain Society produces some excellent materials for both clinicians and patients on its website (www.britishpainsociety.org).

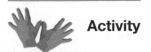 **Activity**

Having read the previous section, answer the following questions. With reference to opioids, what is meant by the terms: 'addiction', 'tolerance' and 'dependence'? To what extent are these likely to occur during the clinical use of opioids for pain relief, and what measures can be taken to minimise these consequences?

Entonox

Entonox, a 50% mixture of oxygen and nitrous oxide, is often overlooked when trying to control acute pain, even though it can be very safe and effective. Nitrous oxide is an analgesic gas that has a fast onset and is excreted rapidly from the body when no longer inhaled. It is able to act so quickly because the tiny molecules cross the capillary walls in the lungs straight into the bloodstream.

As patients hold the mask themselves, Entonox can be considered to be a form of PCA, that is, the patient controls how much gas he or she receives. Entonox is available in portable cylinders for bedside use and comprises a length of tubing with a mask or mouthpiece and a patient demand valve (Figure 4.3). The gas is odourless and colourless; the smell associated with it, which can upset some patients, usually arises from the mask, and can be overcome by using a mouthpiece. When used properly via a close-fitting mask or mouthpiece held in place for at least one minute, analgesia can be maintained. For short painful procedures such as catheterisation, dressing changes, mobilising painful joints and so on, the gas can provide very good pain relief, especially when used in combination with other analgesics. It has been used extensively for labour pain.

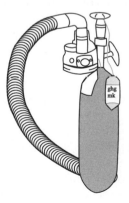

Figure 4.3 Entonox delivery apparatus

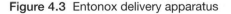

Entonox has proved very valuable for ambulance crews and in A&E, where it is often used to provide pain relief for the simple suturing of wounds and other painful procedures. The gas can even be used to control pain when reducing dislocated fingers or shoulders, provided that the associated muscle spasm is not severe. The gas is extremely safe as there is no drop in blood pressure or serious drop in level of consciousness, although some patients may become drowsy, dizzy or even feel sick. There are a small group of patients who should not receive Entonox. Because nitrous oxide rapidly diffuses into air-filled spaces, it must not be given to patients for whom this may cause problems:

- if **pneumothorax** is suspected or shown
- cases of bowel obstruction
- those with severe head injury
- middle ear and sinus disease
- **decompression sickness**.

Maximising the analgesic prescription

Evidence suggests that there are many missed opportunities, leading to prescribed analgesia not being as potentially effective as it could be (Carr and Thomas 1997; Brockopp et al. 1998; Bucknall et al. 2001; Schafheutle et al. 2001). It is imperative that the nurse takes an active role to ensure that the patient obtains the maximum benefit from their analgesia. The nurse may be faced with an array of analgesics, presenting an ideal opportunity to ensure that the analgesia selected offers 'balanced analgesia' or multimodal pain treatment (Kehlet and Holte 2001), the premise being that total pain relief may not be achieved through the use of a single drug or method without the risk of significant adverse effects. Combining different drugs, such as a NSAID and a centrally acting drug (such as an opioid), offers greater potential pain relief than when the agents are used individually. There is no need to limit this to pharmacological approaches, as combining analgesia and non-pharmacological interventions can optimise pain control by exploiting the multidimensional nature of pain.

The following are examples of some of the potential opportunities to maximise analgesic effectiveness:

- Check the prescription and ensure that the dose and the time interval between doses are correct. Research suggests that doctors frequently underprescribe analgesia and overestimate the dose duration.
- When the dose of analgesia is prescribed as a variable amount, for example 10–20mg, titrate the analgesia against the pain rather than always giving the smallest amount possible.
- Avoid abrupt transitions from parental opioids to non-opioids (Smith 1998). The World Health Organization's (WHO, 1996) analgesic ladder (Figure 4.4) is useful used in reverse to guide analgesic strengths, although be mindful of the evidence on weak opioids.

- When pain is expected to last for at least a few days, consider lobbying for the analgesia to be prescribed on a regular basis for at least 24 hours rather than prn. Around-the-clock dosing is far more effective than traditional prn regimes and ensures analgesia is given before the pain returns.
- Educate patients, their relatives and carers about analgesia and why they should be comfortable, for example to enable them to mobilise and to prevent complications. This will make patients more likely to be open about their pain and to accept analgesia. Better still, get patients even more involved by encouraging them to record their own pain scores and self-administer their analgesia.
- Educate family and friends to ensure that they are aware of the impact on recovery of inadequate pain relief.
- If an opioid has been prescribed, request that an antiemetic and laxative also be ordered, and use these proactively.

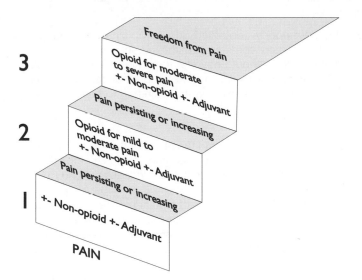

Figure 4.4 The WHO pain ladder
Source: Reproduced with permission from the World Health Organization

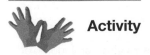 **Activity**

For each of the previous statements, consider the practices and attitudes in your own clinical environment. Make notes on your observations. For example, review the prescription charts and record how many analgesics are prescribed, along with the correct duration of dose. What could feasibly be introduced into your clinical area to improve the administration of analgesia?

Case history

John Moore is a 19-year-old man who was admitted to your ward following a compound fracture of his tibia and fibula. He was given 10mg morphine intravenously in A&E soon after his arrival there. The morphine worked very well, but John found that it was beginning to wear off after about two hours. He was told he would be given more pain relief when he was admitted to a trauma ward very shortly. Because of the general activity level both in A&E and on the ward, three hours elapsed between John's first dose of morphine and the next, which was just 10mg oral morphine syrup. This dose was not titrated to his pain, the inadequate analgesia that this provided was not evaluated and John did not have his pain assessed on a regular basis. The ward was so busy that John only asked for further analgesia when he could stand the pain no longer. Again, because of the workload, this involved a 30-minute delay between his request for urgent pain relief and it being administered.

John continues to have his pain poorly controlled and complains to his family when they come to visit. This is then conveyed to the nurses, who are a bit aggrieved because they feel that John should have let them know earlier that he was in such pain. John, of course, was trying to hide his pain because he was concerned that the nurses were so busy, he felt that his pain had to be really bad for him to trouble them.

Problems illustrated:
- John's pain was not being assessed properly and the effect of the morphine was not evaluated. If this had been done, it would have become obvious that the dose he was receiving was either too small or the time between dosages needed to be reduced.
- He would have benefited from a multimodal regime of regular paracetamol and/or ibuprofen with oral morphine for any breakthrough pain. Patients left in pain that is entirely predictable is common and totally unnecessary even on a busy ward.
- Regular assessment would have encouraged analgesia to be administered before the pain became intolerable.
- Early assessment would have raised the question of whether an opioid alone at a low dose was appropriate, its duration of action for John being only about two hours.
- The original dose was given intravenously to establish analgesia rapidly. However, John is fully able to tolerate oral medication, and oral morphine should have been prescribed for subsequent doses at the time of admission with a dose range of 10–30mg. As John is healthy and had experienced no side effects from the initial dose of intravenous morphine, it would have been quite safe to prescribe this dose 1-hourly prn as long as assessment was done appropriately and pain scores, sedation and respiratory rate recorded.
- Assessment would not only have established that the original oral dose of morphine was inadequate, but also would have indicated that John was going to need regular medication for at least the first 24 hours or until the fracture was fully stabilised.
- A NSAID, which could have been particularly useful for this bone trauma pain, was not prescribed, although there were no contraindications.

Possible solutions:
Routine, regular and ongoing pain assessment would have stopped this situation arising: half-hourly to hourly when initiating analgesia, and then 2-4-hourly to establish effective ongoing pain relief. The use of a regular NSAID such as ibuprofen or diclofenac, commenced in A&E, could well have established analgesia effectively enough to omit or reduce the need for opioids altogether. The regular administration of effective analgesia titrated to the patient's needs and administered during the routine drug round would have been far less distressing for John and also would have reduced the nursing workload.

Patient-controlled analgesia

Patient-controlled analgesia (PCA) is a method of pain control that has been shown to provide more effective pain relief than traditional intramuscular analgesia (Ballantyne et al. 1993). PCA involves patient control of a pump to self-administer analgesia via an intravenous or subcutaneous cannula. The pump is preprogrammed to deliver a small bolus dose of analgesia when the patient presses the button, but a 'lock-out' period prevents the patient receiving further doses should he or she press again within, for example, five minutes.

Several advantages exist for patients. PCA enables them to receive analgesia when they need it, as they do not have to ask a nurse or wait for the nurse to prepare the analgesia. It also avoids the unwanted peaks (leading to sedation, nausea and so on) and troughs (pain) associated with the larger single doses that used to be the case with intramuscular administration. The patient administers small doses, which ensure that the plasma concentration can be kept within a therapeutic level. Although useful for acute pain, PCA is by no means a panacea, as it is not always used to best advantage and does not provide effective enough pain relief following major surgery where an epidural is superior (Schenk et al. 2006; Weber et al. 2007).

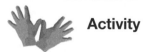 **Activity**

If your ward is currently using PCA, what level of involvement do you have with it? What are the advantages for the patient (ask someone who has used it) and what do staff think of PCA? What are the advantages and disadvantages for them? Consider the wide variety of clinical settings that have used PCA and discuss some of the patient variables, such as locus of control and coping style that may affect the efficacy of PCA.

Research on PCA is very interesting, revealing quite contradictory findings. PCA may not work for all patients as some people do not feel comfortable being responsible for the administration of their own analgesia (Thomas and Rose 1993). Taylor et al. (1996) interviewed patients about using PCA and found negative and positive evaluations, the negative ones including nausea and inadequate analgesia. Koh and Thomas (1994) found that PCA saves nursing time, but according to a Cochrane review (Hudcova et al. 2006), patients receiving PCA are only slightly more satisfied than those receiving traditional analgesia, which is an interesting finding.

Epidural analgesia

Epidural analgesia has become increasingly popular as a method of providing effective pain relief. It is often used postoperatively following major abdominal, thoracic, back or lower limb surgery and during labour. The epidural space is located between the dura mater and the spinal canal. A fine catheter is inserted into the epidural space, between the vertebrae, allowing the delivery of analgesia and local anaesthetics. Figure 4.5 illustrates the location of the needle in the epidural space through which a catheter is threaded to enable continuous drug delivery.

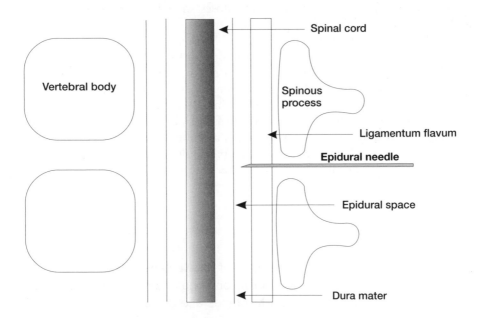

Figure 4.5 Location of needle in epidural space

Opioid drugs can be given in small quantities as they diffuse through the dura mater, binding to opioid receptors in the spinal cord and thus producing analgesia. Local anaesthetic agents such as bupivacaine can also be used, exerting their action by anaesthetising the nerves that enter the spinal cord; this numbs pain in the area supplied by these nerves, for example abdominal wall muscle. There is now overwhelming evidence that epidural analgesia, particularly a thoracic epidural, offers many physiological advantages over other modes of postoperative analgesia, such as a reduced stress response, improved lung function, decreased incidence of pulmonary infections, reduced protein loss and reduced incidence of renal failure (Australian and New Zealand College of Anaesthetists and Faculty of Pain Medicine 2005; Guay 2006). See Chapter 2 for assessment and monitoring protocols.

Nerve blocks

Nerve blocks, once more commonly used to treat chronic pain or aid a diagnosis, are being offered to patients to help treat acute pain. Nerves transmitting pain from a particular organ or body region can be blocked with the injection of a local anaesthetic. Nerve blocks are also used pre-emptively to help prevent subsequent pain from a procedure notorious for resulting in problems such as phantom limb pain following amputation. In older patients for whom hip fractures are common and serious consequences are frequently encountered, the use of a hip block can greatly enhance pain relief without risking the added complications caused by opioid or NSAID use in this vulnerable group (Layzell 2007).

Non-pharmacological approaches to acute pain management

Pain is a multidimensional phenomenon and, as we have already explored (through gate control theory; see Chapter 1), has physical, emotional and cognitive components. It is essential then that effective pain interventions reflect this and that pharmacological interventions are complemented by non-pharmacological approaches administered simultaneously in order to maximise pain control. Many of the interventions used in the management of chronic pain are helpful in the management of acute pain too. Although researching the exact benefit of non-pharmacological strategies can be fraught with problems, given the subjectivity of pain (Sindhu 1996), the reader is referred to Chapter 5 for more information, as well as to an excellent article by Stevenson (1995), which, although a little dated, still gives a good overview.

The following interventions have been selected as they are becoming more widely used in acute pain, but this is only an introduction to a fascinating field of pain management.

Psychological preparation and information-giving

Prior to any potentially painful procedure, patients indicate that effective information provision and psychological preparation are helpful and can reduce anxiety (Gilmartin and Wright 2007). Bandolier's review (1999) goes as far as to state that preoperative interventions, which combine sensory and procedural information, significantly reduce postoperative pain, distress and negative effects. Preparing patients for surgery and potential pain is becoming increasingly important as more and more patients experience surgery in day case units or short stay facilities where they will be discharged shortly after surgery and will need to take responsibility for their own pain management quickly and effectively. Although this can be vital in preparing patients for surgery or for a painful procedure, a sensitive approach will be needed for some patients who use denial as a coping strategy. However, most people welcome the opportunity to obtain as much information as possible to help them prepare, feel confident and in control (Gilmartin 2007). In most cases, the ideal is to give verbal information initially and then follow this up in written form. Most patients do not appear to recall much of what is told them prior to surgery or a painful procedure as their mind is occupied just considering these potentially stressful events.

Massage

It is thought that, by stimulating the skin, the large diameter A beta fibres can be activated, which then close the 'pain gate' and prevent pain impulses from C fibres reaching the central nervous system. Gentle firm stroking of the foot, hand or arm is often a very effective relaxation intervention for pain relief and can easily be used while waiting for analgesia to take effect or during a procedure. Family and friends often feel helpless when seeing a loved one in pain but simple massage or gentle stroking can bring comfort and also help them to feel needed.

Relaxation

Psychological strategies are widely used for the reduction of distress and anxiety by reducing muscle tension, encouraging an inner sense of calm and diminishing the activity of the autonomic nervous system. They should be used in addition to pharmacological interventions. Pain often produces anxiety, which in turn produces muscle tension and more pain. Breaking the cycle using relaxation techniques is an important way of reducing the pain or helping the person to cope with his or her pain.

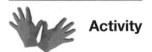 **Activity**

The next time you are with patients who have been experiencing pain, ask them whether they find any strategies other than medication useful. Ask them what they do to help themselves relax when they feel tense. Make notes on this and on the effectiveness of any of the strategies they mention.

Deep breathing strategies, such as counting up to 10 slowly and then back again as one exhales, focus on breathing and reduce tension and anxiety. Music can be used as a relaxation or distraction strategy in pain management. In a recent Cochrane review of music therapy, Cepeda et al. (2004) found that music reduced pain, increased the number of patients who reported at least 50% pain relief and reduced requirements for strong opioid analgesia. Using a personal stereo, the volume can be increased or decreased in response to the pain. Patients can be encouraged to bring their favourite music into hospital. Remember to suggest music in the community, especially if an unpleasant dressing change needs to be undertaken in a person's home, as this strategy can reinforce a multimodal approach to pain relief.

Distraction

Distraction is a strategy that allows one's mind to focus on pleasant stimuli rather than on pain or negative emotions (McCaffery and Beebe 1994). Patients who experience chronic pain routinely use distraction strategies, but they can be helpful for reducing acute pain also. They can range from watching television or reading a book, to more physical pursuits such as going for a walk. Most people have developed their own distraction activities to help them to cope with pain, but when they need to go to hospital, they might feel unable, or even forget, to use some of these useful techniques.

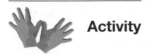 **Activity**

Ask four patients whether they use anything to distract themselves from pain when they are at home. If they have ever been admitted to hospital, did they successfully employ these strategies while they were in hospital? If not, how could they be incorporated into their care?

Comfort

Comfort is often forgotten as an actual intervention for pain control. It is important to note here that these strategies may be particularly helpful with people who have learning disabilities or senile dementia. The inability to express one's pain must only contribute to the fear and dread of its getting worse. Comfort strategies can include positioning, the presence of family and friends, and the skilled companionship of nursing staff.

Skilled companionship

Nurses may avoid patients who are experiencing pain or display 'blocking' behaviour if they feel that there is nothing they can do or it makes them feel awkward and uncomfortable (Booth et al. 1996). Blocking behaviour describes strategies that healthcare professionals use when they wish to avoid inquiring about the social and emotional impact of pain or illness for fear that it will increase patients' distress, take up too much time, or impact on their own emotional survival. Consequently, they may offer reassurance before the main problems have been identified, explain away distress as normal, attend to physical needs only, switch the topic or just try to 'jolly' patients along (Maguire and Pitceathly 2002).

When pain is distressing, the close company of another person can help the sufferer to cope with the experience. Nurses can stay with the person and just be there for them. When nurses have stayed with patients at this time, patients talk about the nurse 'knowing what I was going through' or say, 'I just knew that they were there and it helped me cope.' Holding the person, letting him or her talk and just sitting quietly are all important actions that should be part of the rich repertoire of nursing care. We should not fear another's pain or suffering but allow ourselves to enter their world and be there for them.

Case history

Mrs Peters has a venous leg ulcer, which requires daily visits by the community nurse. The dressing change is often difficult as the dressing sticks to the exudate and tissue beneath. The nurses ask Mrs Peters to take some analgesics an hour before they come but this is often ineffective as they arrive too early or too late. Each time Mrs Peters tries to hold her winces and small yelps of pain at bay, as she doesn't want to hurt the feelings of the nurse. She knows they don't mean to cause her such pain. The nurses find the whole process very distressing and try and get it over as quickly as possible, which usually results in more pain.

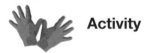 **Activity**

Look around your ward, department or in the community. Do we make it easy for patients to use non-pharmacological strategies? If in hospital, can patients see outside to watch the sky and trees? Are there televisions and radios available, or can their relatives bring them in? Are there telephones by the beds so that patients may talk to their friends and relatives? Are visiting times fairly generous? Do you have enough skilled staff to be able to ensure comfort and skilled companionship?

Some of these things may not seem terribly relevant, but if you have pain that is difficult to control, access to some or all of the above can make a significant difference. If patients are being nursed in a far from ideal environment, and away from their home comforts, as nurses we should be able to articulate the benefits of some of these far from obvious pain-relieving strategies. Patient studies often cite the more esoteric as being of great value, but we lose sight of this in the hubbub of a district general hospital. Palliative care units, however, have been successful in emphasising the benefits of environment, comfort and distraction.

Transcutanous electrical nerve stimulation

Transcutaneous electrical nerve stimulation (TENS) is mentioned here, although it is covered in more detail in Chapter 5 on chronic pain. It is a non-invasive method that has been used for acute pain and for women in labour. Like many complementary therapies, so far the research to support its use is not robust, although certain patients do appear to derive benefit. The apparatus consists of a small electrical pulse generator, the size of a personal stereo, with two or four electrodes that are placed on the skin (see Figure 4.6). It is battery powered, and the electrical impulse discharged can be altered in intensity, duration and frequency for each individual. It is suggested that the electrical stimulation excites the larger diameter A beta fibres and closes the 'pain gate', as well as stimulating the release of endorphins (Walsh 1997). The TENS machine can easily be worn beneath clothes and does not restrict mobility, which allows the patient to continue normal activities such as work or gardening.

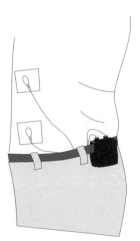

Figure 4.6 A TENS machine attached to a patient's belt with electrodes on the body

Conclusion

This chapter has encouraged you to critically reflect on the current management of acute pain. It has utilised pharmacological and non-pharmacological strategies that reflect the multidimensional nature of pain in order to plan effective pain interventions. In practice, the approach to acute pain management might incorporate only pharmacological interventions, and it is essential to consider broader approaches. By reflecting on your own practice and that of your colleagues, it is possible to increase considerably the diversity of approaches being used. Encompassing the perspective of the patient will help to facilitate effective intervention and improve patient care.

It should be considered that the poor or inappropriate management of acute pain could well lead to the development of chronic benign pain. This is particularly the case with chronic low back pain, which will be covered in more depth in Chapter 5. Chronic low back pain was recognised as one of the most common and costly health problems in Western societies in the late twentieth century (Linton 1994), even more alarming perhaps when one considers the statement by Waddell (1992), a leading professor in orthopaedic surgery, that most chronic back pain is the **iatrogenic** consequence of inappropriate medical advice. This is undoubtedly food for thought as we attempt to relieve acute pain more effectively.

After a break, try the multiple choice test below in order to self-assess your understanding so far. For some of the questions, more than one answer will be correct, however, there will be one answer that is so far best supported by the evidence.

Suggested further reading

Counsell D. and Pediani R. (2004) *Patient Controlled Epidural Analgesia*. Oxford, Butterworth-Heinemann.

Evidence-based Perioperative Medicine, Geneva (2004) *Systematic Reviews in Anaesthesia, Analgesia and Critical Care*, http://www.hcuge.ch/anesthesie/anglais/evidence/arevusyst.htm#top.

Gan T., Woolf C., Brennan T., Kehlet H. and Mekhail N. (2004) Unraveling the mechanisms and clinical consequences of pain: recent discoveries and the implications for pain management. *Medscape*, http://www.medscape.com/pages/public/about/about.

Gruener D. (2004) New strategies for managing acute pain episodes in patients with chronic pain. *Medscape*, http://www.medscape.com/pages/public/about/about.

Harmer M. (2002) *Patient-controlled Analgesia*. Oxford, Blackwell Science.

Macintyre P. and Schug S. (2007) *Acute Pain Management: A Practical Guide*, 3rd edn. Edinburgh, Saunders Elsevier.

Middleton C. (2006) *Epidural Analgesia in Acute Pain Management*. Hoboken, NJ, John Wiley & Sons.

Park G., Fulton B. and Senturan S. (2006) *The Management of Acute Pain*. Oxford, Oxford Medical Publications.

Scottish Intercollegiate Guidelines Network (2004) *Post Operative Management in Adults: A Practical to Postoperative Care for Clinical Staff*, http://www.sign.ac.uk/pdf/sign77.pdf.

Sherwood G., McNeill J., Starck P. and Disnard G. (2003) Changing acute pain management outcomes in surgical patients: research. *AORN Journal*, http://www.findarticles.com/p/articles/mi_m0FSL/is_2_77/ai_98134862.

Managing Acute Pain
Multiple choice TEST

1. Which of the following side effects of pain and stress are most likely to contribute specifically to immunosuppression and increased risk of infection?
   a. Atelectasis ☐
   b. Increased platelet adhesion ☐
   c. Increased metabolic rate ☐
   d. Nausea ☐

2. Which of the following is a pain-producing substance that is blocked by treatment with NSAIDs?
   a. Prostaglandin ☐
   b. Prothrombin ☐
   c. Prostacyclin ☐
   d. Prolactin ☐

3. Which of the following drugs is particularly useful for treating inflammatory pain?
   a. Paracetamol ☐
   b. Codeine ☐
   c. NSAIDs ☐
   d. Diamorphine ☐

4. How are opioids thought to relieve pain?
   a. By reducing inflammation ☐
   b. By acting at the site of tissue damage ☐
   c. By blocking pain signals in the central nervous system ☐
   d. By making the patient sleep ☐

5. Which of the following is not a common side effect of opioids?
   a. Sedation ☐
   b. Nausea and vomiting ☐
   c. Constipation ☐
   d. Respiratory depression ☐

6. Which is the safest route by which to administer a titrated dose of opioid?
   a. Orally ☐
   b. Intramuscularly ☐
   c. Intravenously ☐
   d. Rectally ☐

7. Which statement most accurately describes how strategies such as massage and TENS work?
   a. They distract the patient from thinking about their pain ☐
   b. They work by exciting the nerve fibres and opening the pain gate ☐
   c. They stimulate the release of prostaglandins ☐
   d. They excite the A beta fibres and close the pain gate ☐

8. Which of the following most accurately describes a distraction strategy in the context of pain management?
   a. Thinking of a nice holiday and visualising yourself there ☐

> b. Slowly counting to 10 while breathing in, and then slowly exhaling □
> c. Watching television □
> d. Listening to a piano concerto by Brahms □
>
> 9. Which of the following patients should not receive Entonox?
>   a. Those experiencing a heart attack □
>   b. A pregnant woman □
>   c. A patient in renal failure □
>   d. A patient with a head injury □
>
> 10. Which of the following analgesics should not be given together?
>   a. Paracetamol and a NSAID □
>   b. A NSAID and morphine □
>   c. Codeine and buprenorphine □
>   d. Aspirin and paracetamol □

Answers

1. c. Metabolic rate is particularly implicated in immunosuppression. All the others are unpleasant and potentially dangerous side effects of pain and stress but have not so far been specifically linked to depression of the immune system.

2. a. Prostaglandin E is the end product of a chain of chemical events that results once tissue damage has occurred. It is known to increase the activity of the nerves conducting pain impulses and therefore exacerbates the pain. Prothrombin is an inactive substance in blood plasma that is the precursor of thrombin, which clots the blood. Prostacyclin is a type of prostaglandin produced by the endothelial lining of the blood vessels; it inhibits platelet aggregation, thus reducing the blood clotting time. Prolactin is the pituitary hormone that initiates lactation.

3. c. NSAIDs; tissue damage following surgery results in a prostaglandin release, which is implicated in the development and maintenance of inflammation.

4. c. By blocking pain signals in the central nervous system. More recent research also indicates that opioids have some action on the peripheral nervous system. NSAIDs reduce inflammation and also act at the site of tissue damage. Opioids can make patients feel sleepy, but this is incidental to their pain-relieving properties.

5. d. Respiratory depression is quite unusual when opioids are used correctly: it is very rare for opioids to induce respiratory depression once a patient has taken opioids for a few days. Sedation is quite common when opioids are used for the first time. Nausea and vomiting affect about 30% of opioid users during the first few days of use, and constipation causes potential problems for the majority of opioid users.

6. c. Intravenously; this route is the safest, as the onset of action is less than one minute and the peak effect (including unwanted side effects) can usually be seen after seven minutes. With oral administration, the onset of action can be anywhere between five minutes and one hour. Uptake from intramuscular injection is also variable (5–70 minutes), being influenced by such things as hydration, cold and hypotension.

7. d. They excite the A beta fibres and close the pain gate, thus reducing the perception of pain. It is suggested that they may also encourage the release of endorphins.

8. c. Watching television is a distraction as it channels thoughts away from the pain. Although all the strategies involve a degree of distraction, thinking back to a nice holiday is usually part of 'guided imagery' and is a cognitive strategy (that is, it modifies thought processes) used in the management of pain. Distraction and imagery are both cognitive strategies. Deep breathing and listening to a relaxing piece of music are both behavioural strategies that modify the physiological reaction to pain.

9. d. A patient with a head injury because of the potential to raise intracranial pressure. Patients with all the other conditions should be able to tolerate Entonox safely for short periods.

10. c. Codeine and buprenorphine should not be given together. They are both opioids, codeine is a weak mu agonist and buprenorphine an agonist/antagonist. All the others are perfectly safe given together and can form part of multimodal analgesia.

CHAPTER 5

Managing Chronic Pain

Learning outcomes

On completion of this chapter, the student will be able to:

■ Briefly analyse contemporary theory of the development and maintenance of chronic pain

■ Review the pharmaceutical, psychological, behavioural, social and physical strategies used in the management of chronic pain

■ Critically discuss professional collaboration in the holistic management of the person experiencing chronic pain

■ Analyse practices for managing chronic pain in his or her own clinical area and identify methods of influencing change

Indicative reading

Ashburn, M. and Staats P. (1999) Management of chronic pain. *Lancet*, **353**: 1865–9.

Bandolier (2007) Chronic non-malignant pain, http://www.jr2.ox.ac.uk/bandolier/booth/painpag/chronic.html.

DIPEx.org., Personal Experiences of Health and Illness, Chronic Pain, http://www.dipex.org/chronicpain.

Gatchel R., Peng Y., Peters M., Fuchs P. and Turk D. (2007) The biopsychosocial approach to chronic pain: scientific advances and future directions. *Psychological Bulletin*, **133**(4): 581–624.

Main C. and Williams A. (2002) Clinical reviews. ABC of psychological medicine. Musculoskeletal pain. *British Medical Journal*, **325**: 534–7, www.bmj.bmjjournals.com.

Pither C., Cognitive behavioural approaches to chronic pain, http://www.wellcome.ac.uk/en/pain/microsite/medicine3.html.

Shaw S. (2006) Nursing and supporting patients with chronic pain. *Nursing Standard*, **20**(19): 60–5.

Wells C., Chronic pain management, http://www.thepainweb.com/doclib/topics/000006.htm#drugs.

Background

Begin by reading some of the literature cited in the indicative reading section above. This will provide an understanding of some of the current theories about the development of chronic pain as well as interventions for management and some of the issues and barriers that impede progress. Contemporary research is beginning to provide us with possible explanations as to why chronic pain may develop in the first place, as well as suggesting some answers as to why effective management can remain so elusive.

Chronic pain has been defined as pain that lasts continuously or intermittently for three months or more (IASP 1986). Although it is always neat to have a definition like this, a specific time frame is increasingly being questioned, with the recognition that an acute pain that does not resolve with tissue healing potentially becomes problematic at a much earlier stage. Waddell (1992) suggested that acute back pain, for example, if treated inappropriately, can become chronic within days of its onset. Chronic pain can be further categorised as being either 'malignant' or 'non-malignant' (this is also sometimes called persistent pain). It is important to distinguish between the two, as the approach to treatment is different. Chronic non-malignant pain is persistent and has no end point. McCaffery and Beebe (1989, p. 232) define chronic non-malignant pain as:

> pain that has lasted 6 months or longer, is ongoing on a daily basis, is due to non-threatening causes, has not responded to currently available treatment methods, and may continue for the remainder of the patient's life.

Where chronic pain lacks a specific organic and curable cause, the philosophy of treatment usually focuses on helping patients to take responsibility for their pain and helping them to cope with it using a variety of strategies. Reducing the consumption of ineffective analgesia, challenging negative beliefs and inappropriate coping strategies, rehabilitation, increasing function and improving quality of life are common goals of treatment. In contrast, chronic malignant pain may have an end point with its relationship to a terminal illness. Treatment approaches include analgesia that is given in sufficient amount to relieve the pain and at doses not normally considered for non-malignant pain. Treatment goals also include symptom control, as well as other strategies reflecting the multidimensional nature of pain.

Given the different approaches to the two types of chronic pain, this chapter will only consider chronic non-malignant pain, although many of the non-pharmacological approaches are equally helpful for chronic malignant pain. Pain associated with malignant disease is a subject in itself and readers are recommended to access the CD-ROM 'Breaking Barriers: Management of Cancer-related Pain' developed by the Institute for Cancer Research in collaboration with the Royal Marsden Hospital (2008).

The following section explores some of the possible explanations for chronic pain as well as considering the experience of chronic pain from the patient's perspective. We will then go on to consider a range of strategies to help to manage chronic pain in the context of its possible cause, discussing pharmacological and non-pharmacological interventions. Finally, the importance of collaboration with patients, healthcare professionals, family, carers and even employers is emphasised if meaningful improvements in pain management and quality of life are going to be sustained.

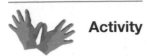 **Activity**

Before starting the following section, visit http://www.dipex.org/chronicpain. There are 47 interviews with people who have chronic pain across a range of ages. It explores their experiences and also how their pain has been treated. There are also informative explanations about the conditions. Choose a couple of people and listen to their stories.

What is chronic non-malignant or persistent pain?

Although it is helpful to think about what types of disease might generate chronic pain, it is also important to consider what might be generating or maintaining pain in the absence of an identifiable organic cause.

Potential pathological pain generators

For disease processes such as rheumatoid arthritis, ongoing inflammation seems to be the obvious cause and for many the pattern will be one of flare-ups of pain followed by periods when pain may subside. Sufferers of chronic headaches such as migraine will again experience flare-ups followed by periods of being pain free but are still regarded as sufferers of chronic pain.

Neuropathic pain can be a feature of acute, chronic malignant and chronic non-malignant pain and is caused by damage to nerves from diseases such as diabetes, MS and **Parkinson's disease**. Nerves may also be damaged during surgery, following trauma or virus infection, even from nutritional deficits and toxins such as alcohol. Nerve injury can then be the starting point for reactive changes that sweep centrally to produce abnormal neural function (Kehlet et al. 2006). Neuropathic pain has been described as pain related to abnormal processing within the nervous system. The International Association for the Study of Pain defines it as 'pain initiated or caused by a primary lesion or dysfunction of the nervous system' (Merskey and Bogduk 1994). It has also been described as pain as a consequence of injury or disease affecting the peripheral and/or central nervous systems associated with various sensory and/or motor phenomena (Backonja 2003). Neuropathic pain continues beyond the normal period of tissue healing and is associated with serious co-morbidity and major disability (Cavenagh et al. 2006; Gustorff et al. 2008). Nerve damage can change the biochemistry and anatomic circuitry of primary sensory afferents as well as spinal and brain neurones. The field of neuropathic pain is a relatively new area of scientific discovery, which is opening up new and revised forms of treatment quite different from the usual drug and treatment regimes for non-neuropathic pain (Rolke et al. 2006). Unfortunately, evidence suggests that healthcare professionals continue to treat neuropathic pain as they would nociceptive pain and this may contribute to the failure of many patients to obtain improved pain control. The treatment of neuropathic pain will be briefly covered in this chapter but for more in-depth information, please refer to the suggested further reading section.

Other causes of chronic pain include any form of ischaemia (**angina** or **intermittent claudication**, for example). Chronic obstructive airways disease can cause chest pain. But why do some people experience inflammatory disease, nerve injury, ischaemia and so on and experience unremitting and distressing pain, while others with similar conditions do not? Alternatively, why do some individuals report quite significant levels of chronic pain with seemingly little impact, as they are able to lead full and active lives? An analysis of 1,000 consultations in general practice revealed that 11.3% were for a pain of more than three months' duration (Potter 1990).

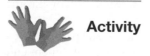 **Activity**

Think of some more causes of chronic non-malignant pain. Ask people whether they experience continuous pain.

The causes of pain appear to be far more complex than we first thought and our initial attempts to combat chronic pain from a biomedical perspective were nearly always doomed to failure. The bottom line is that we all experience pain against a complex physiological, genetic and psychosocial background and it is the interplay of these factors that influence the conversion of a sensory activity into a pain experience, requiring it to be viewed from a biopsychosocial perspective.

Case history

David is a carpenter with a large building firm. He is married with two teenage children. His wife works locally in retail but travels extensively to Southeast Asia sourcing new lines for the business. Six months ago David was lifting some boxes when his 'back went'. He took a week off work and stayed in bed, hoping it would get better and anxious not to harm his back further. Although he returned to work, the pain has continued. He has seen his GP who has diagnosed a simple non-specific back strain but has referred him to an orthopaedic surgeon. David feels restricted by the constant aching pain and is irritable with the family. He is anxious that the pain will never go away and he will not be able to continue working. His life feels a shadow of its former vibrancy.

Reflect on David's situation. What do you think he feels and why? Make notes and then read the following section.

There are many possible generators for maintaining chronic pain. This is a hugely complex area, so for more in-depth information, please refer to the suggested further reading. Pain generators include:

- *Neuronal plasticity.* We covered this briefly in earlier chapters especially when we explored inflammatory pain, which we usually expect to resolve spontaneously. However, unlike the temporary hyperalgesia produced by inflammation, stimulation of peripheral nerves can, in some individuals, produce persistent abnormal neurobiological changes leading to chronic pain.
- *Genetic factors.* Sensitivity to clinical pain differs considerably, as no two individuals will report the same experience. It is now widely accepted that genetic factors influence susceptibility to the generation and experience of chronic pain as well as the response to analgesia.
- *Previous pain*: This correlates well with the development of certain chronic neuropathic pain, for example severe and painful shingles often precedes a severe case of **postherpetic neuralgia**. There also appears to be a correlation in certain individuals between severe uncontrolled postoperative pain and the increased risk of chronic pain as a consequence.
- *Psychosocial factors.* Particularly in the case of chronic musculoskeletal pain, psychological, social and economic factors play a significant part in the development and maintenance of chronic pain (Turk and Okifuji 1996). Expectation of pain, levels of distress, fear, depression, pessimism, avoidance of activity, past memories, social environment, work satisfaction and levels of physical activity can all impact on the course of chronic pain. There is also work being undertaken on the negative impact of stress, anger, sleep deprivation and childhood abuse. Perceived control and self-efficacy appear to be important, as individuals shown to have high self-efficacy generally display a greater motivation to engage in health-promoting behaviours and better adherence to treatment. Self-efficacy even appears to affect the body's immune and opioid systems (Weisenberg 1998). Vulnerability or resilience and certain personality traits have also been implicated in chronic pain development. Temperament and personality may predispose some people to make certain kinds of maladaptive appraisals to situations, while others will be more resilient. Research also suggests that exposure to severe stressors and how we react to them not only changes neurobiological processes and structures, negatively impacting on thresholds for pain, but also potentially reduces our ability to cope with subsequent stress.

Reflecting back on the previous case study and David's plight, you will see links between his situation and some of the factors above. In particular, his worry and anxiety about the future and how this may impact upon his own management of the pain. His initial response was to stay inactive and it appears he hasn't done much to help himself. This may be related to 'fear avoidance', which is often associated with those experiencing back pain (Pincus et al. 2006). Early detection of such concerns is important to prevent long-term pain and disability.

• *Physical deconditioning:* Although we still lack research to entirely support the impact of physical deconditioning, that is, the loss of physical fitness through illness or lack of exercise (Smeets and Wittink 2007), for many years pain management programmes have worked on improving physical function in chronic pain sufferers, particularly those with musculoskeletal pain. It is posited that pain limits activity through fear avoidance and this can lead to deconditioning-related physiological changes, such as muscle atrophy, changes in metabolism, **osteoporosis** and obesity, as well as functional changes, such as a decrease in cardiovascular capacity, a decrease in muscle strength and impaired motor control. At the very least, improving levels of fitness could be thought to impact on endorphins, weight gain and feelings of self-esteem, which can only be beneficial.

• *Age and gender:* It is early days yet but research is beginning to show differences in how gender and age may influence the development of chronic pain.

The impact of the above factors illustrates that chronic pain does not fit the biomedical model on which so much of our diagnosis and treatment hinged. A biopsychosocial model is more helpful but will take time to influence clinical treatment and patient perception. Patients particularly have been shown to strongly hold the belief that pain always has an 'organic' cause and they can emphatically reject psychological factors as an explanation, which can severely limit effective treatment strategies and a positive outcome (Eccleston et al. 1997; Walsh and Radcliffe 2002; Allcock et al. 2007).

The patient's perspective: experiencing chronic pain

Let us now explore pain from the patient's perspective. Before we do this, however, it would be helpful for you to carry out the following activity.

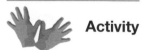 **Activity**

Select two patients within your clinical area who suffer from a chronic painful condition. Ask them to tell you as much about their pain as possible. To do this, it is necessary to be fairly unstructured, as you want them to talk 'openly' and give you plenty of information. However, questions might include:

Tell me about your pain. Where is it? When did it start? How long has it lasted? How intense is it? What does the pain feel like? Note, for example, the words that patients use to describe their pain, such as ache, stabbing and shooting.

What helps your pain? What makes it worse? How does the pain affect the quality of your life? Do you have difficulty sleeping? Does the pain wake you at night? Does it affect your mood and appetite? What could the nurses do to make your pain better or help you to cope with it? Do you take any medication for your pain? Do you have any side effects from the medication? Do you use any coping strategies, for example relaxation? How do your family feel about your pain?

Each interview should take 20–30 minutes. Recording it will save you having to take notes (but always ask the patient's permission first). Otherwise, write down as much as you can. Also include your observations of the patient (facial expressions, body language and so on).

Time out

Reflect on the findings from your interview. What are the implications for your practice? From the information you have obtained, are there features that would be valuable for colleagues to know? Does your clinical area have mechanisms in place for communicating some of your findings, such as a pain assessment tool in the care plan?

Many studies have explored the experiences of people with chronic pain and found that pain adversely affected many dimensions of their lives. Most studies found that the most important factor for patients was that their pain was believed; when you spoke with your patients about their chronic pain, they might have mentioned this to you. Being listened to, for someone to understand and show that they understand the pain that patients are experiencing are significant issues, especially when there has been no formal diagnosis. When no satisfactory explanation for pain has been forthcoming, patients may become preoccupied with trying to discover the cause. No explanation helps to fuel fears that they will not be believed, and that their pain is 'all in the mind' – increasing their distress and frustration. Many patients need reassurance that their pain is real, and need a diagnosis or explanation of their pain to provide 'legitimacy' for their suffering and their 'sick role'. It seems a universal experience of all suffers of chronic pain that they feel those around them – family, friends, employers and healthcare professionals – question the authenticity of their pain experience (Allcock et al. 2007).

For any care to begin to be meaningful, it needs to reflect the psychosocial and cultural context of chronic pain and the impact that patients' backgrounds or social environments may have on how they respond to and cope with chronic pain. So many factors are known to influence how much distress pain will cause an individual. We all probably know of people who seem to cope with intolerable levels of pain with little if any obvious impact on the quality of their lives or the enjoyment of their social interactions. Other individuals, however, become entirely consumed by pain; they constantly seek input from healthcare professionals in a desperate bid to have their pain explained. These unfortunate individuals will often have massive medical files as they are referred to doctor after doctor in a usually fruitless attempt to find a 'cure'.

Managing chronic pain

Before we consider some of the strategies that can be used, it is helpful to review how chronic pain is managed in your area. You will need to spend some time on this; the following activities are suggested to enable you to explore this aspect more fully.

 Time out

Think back to those patients who could be identified as experiencing chronic pain. Glance at some assessments and care plans – is their pain documented? Apart from a pain assessment tool, how else might you obtain information from patients about their pain?

The underdocumentation of pain is well reported (Dalton et al. 2001), but documentation provides an important role in the management of pain as it allows us to share information and evaluate the effectiveness of interventions.

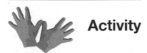 **Activity**

List all the interventions that are used to manage chronic pain in your clinical practice, maybe bracketing them into pharmacological and non-pharmacological strategies. Identify how each intervention relates to contemporary theories of pain perception. Do the interventions reflect the multidimensional nature of pain, that is, are multiple strategies incorporated into pain management, or are single pharmacological strategies the only ones made explicit?

All too often, healthcare professionals do not explore patients' views on their pain management, instead focusing on biomedical and pharmacological interventions. Strategies such as increasing knowledge about how and why chronic pain may develop, identifying and treating depression, challenging maladaptive coping, improving self-esteem, tackling poor sleeping patterns, increasing functional capacity and general fitness can all contribute to the reduction of pain or help patients to 'cope' with their pain better. Given that pain is multidimensional, it is logical that patients will benefit from a range of different approaches. The next section explores some of the pharmacological approaches to chronic pain and the use of pharmacological and non-pharmacological interventions.

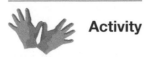 **Activity**

Review the care plans relating to a problem of pain for three patients. Are the problems clearly stated? Are the goals realistic, measurable, achievable and patient centred? Are the interventions all documented? Have the care plans been evaluated? Write the results up in table format.

What are your thoughts on your findings? You may be surprised to find how little is documented about the main symptom that first brought the patients into contact with their doctor or your area of clinical practice.

Pharmacological approaches to pain management

Drug therapy can be an important part of treatment, and the reader is referred to Chapter 4 to review the main analgesics. In chronic (and acute) pain, analgesia and adjuvant drug therapies are often used alongside other interventions, depending on what is appearing to drive and maintain the pain. However, many treatment plans encourage patients to reduce their consumption of analgesia and focus on coping strategies, reserving analgesia, if it has proved effective in the past, for acute exacerbations. For many chronic pain sufferers, simple analgesia such as paracetamol and NSAIDs or weak opioids no longer work. If pain responds to strong opioid analgesia, the doses may need to be quite high and the side effects unacceptable. People often need to learn how to live with their pain and minimise the discomfort. Having said that, there are, however, examples of chronic non-malignant pain that do respond reasonably well to specific medication. Although the range of drugs has not greatly increased over the past 10 years or so, how some of these drugs are administered has changed substantially. To avoid problems associated with oral medications, far more preparations now are available as topical agents, in patch format, for example fentanyl and buprenorphine patches, or are administered via implantable devices delivering drugs intrathecally via a catheter implanted into the back. The types of medication used for chronic pain other than simple analgesia will now be explored in more detail.

Adjuvant drug therapy

Adjuvant therapy describes drugs that do not have an obvious analgesic action but can, because of the complex origins of some types of pain, provide relief in certain conditions and circumstances. The exact action of some of these drugs is unknown. They can be given alone or alongside traditional analgesia to improve pain relief: several will now be considered in a little more detail.

Antidepressants

These drugs seem to provide analgesia by enhancing neurotransmitter activity at the terminals in the pain-modulating pathways. These are the pathways that originate in the brain and help the nervous system to tone down the incoming pain signals. Amitriptyline is one such drug often used to treat chronic neuropathic pain and some of the newer antidepressants are showing promise, with a slightly better side effect profile. The dose given is usually much lower than that given to treat depression. When the drug is given to treat depression, the patient's response or improvement may take some time. When antidepressants are given to enhance pain relief, however, some patients appear to respond quite quickly. Even though the doses may be low, analgesia may also be enhanced because patients experience some antidepressant action. Antidepressants can sedate so some patients will also find that they can get to sleep a little easier, especially when the drug is given at night.

If the dose has to be increased in order to achieve a response, patients must be informed of the side effects of these drugs, which may include sedation, constipation, a dry mouth and dizziness. At the low doses given for patients in pain, serious side effects are rare although the elderly are more commonly adversely affected. For further information, see Mico et al. (2006) or McQuay (2004).

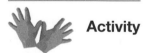 **Activity**

Think about how a patient might feel after visiting the GP for chronic pain and being prescribed an antidepressant. What information would the patient also need to receive?

Patients with chronic pain frequently become very demoralised. Many will have undergone a battery of diagnostic tests that prove negative – but they still continue to have pain. When antidepressants are prescribed, the patient may feel that the doctor thinks it is 'all in my head' and does not really believe the pain. It is essential to explain that the antidepressant is thought to work on chemicals in the brain to reduce pain and is not being used to improve mood, as the dose involved is very different. It is equally important to recognise that many people with chronic pain will be depressed; successful management requires great sensitivity and understanding.

Anticonvulsants

These drugs provide analgesia for the shooting pains that occur with nerve damage. Like most of the drugs described here, their mechanism of action is not fully understood. It is thought that carbamazepine and phenytoin stabilise abnormal nerve firing as they do for patients experiencing convulsions. Carbamazepine has been found to be particularly useful for treating trigeminal neuralgia. Unfortunately, some patients suffer dizziness, epigastric pain, nausea and drowsiness. The newer anticonvulsants such as gabapentin and pregabalin are prescribed for the treatment of chronic neuropathic pain and appear to have fewer side effects. They may even have some utility when used pre-emptively to treat acute pain. Synergism has been shown to exist with gabapentin and morphine, suggesting that, when given perioperatively, oral gabapentin may decrease pain scores in the early postoperative period as well as morphine consumption and associated side effects (Turan et al. 2004).

Antispasmodic agents

Baclofen is a substance used to treat smooth muscle spasm but can be effective in treating spasm caused by severe nerve damage, especially in spasticity (Stempien and Tsai 2000). The principal side effects are sedation, confusion and muscle weakness. Buscopan can be useful for relieving abdominal spasm for chronically painful conditions such as irritable bowel syndrome (IBS) (Zuccaroli and Van Schoor 2007).

Antihypertensives

Clonidine is a central and peripheral alpha-adrenergic blocker and can be an effective analgesic for certain conditions including neuropathic pain, although its utility is limited by sedation and hypotension. Its use in a patch may prove useful for certain conditions in the future.

Steroids

These drugs are used quite frequently for the pain caused by a chronic inflammatory condition that has suddenly got worse. They are also used extensively when injected into joints to help relieve conditions such as back pain and arthritis of the hip and for patients suffering with advanced cancer pain. The drugs work in a variety of ways but probably provide analgesia by reducing the oedema that may be pressing on nerves or pain-sensitive structures. Their anti-inflammatory effects may also reduce the levels of the pain-producing chemicals found in damaged tissues. Steroids are not to be confused with non-steroidal anti-inflammatory drugs (NSAIDs), which are analgesic drugs particularly useful for treating acute inflammatory pain. NSAIDs are used in chronic pain management to treat an acute flare-up of a chronic inflammatory condition such as arthritis but appear to have little or no effect on chronic neuro-pathic pain.

Muscle relaxants: benzodiazepines

These drugs, for example diazepam, are more commonly used to control acute musc-uloskeletal pain, particularly low back pain where there is muscle spasm. They are not appropriate for long-term use because of their addiction potential. Diazepam has been shown to bring pain relief for patients with a high level of anxiety or insomnia.

Ketamine

Ketamine is thought to exert its analgesic effect by antagonism of the NMDA recep-tor complex, which is implicated in pain 'wind-up'. The drug is a general anaesthetic but also has a strong analgesic action. It can, however, cause severe dysphoria (the opposite of euphoria) and terrible nightmares or dreams when used in anaesthetic doses. Ketamine may be tried in sub-anaesthetic doses when a patient is not obtain-ing relief from large doses of opioids, but its side effects mean that it is usually reserved for 'difficult' cases. It is only available as a parenteral preparation and should therefore be given as a low-dose infusion, although some recent studies have been conducted indicating it can be useful when the parenteral preparation is given orally. See Chapter 4 on the use of ketamine perioperatively to potentially reduce the risks of chronic pain development following surgery.

Capsaicin

This is a substance derived from chilli peppers and has been used for a variety of conditions particularly neuropathic pain. Capsaicin is applied as a cream and is thought to deplete local sensory nerve terminals of substance P. Because capsaicin causes irritation of the skin, blind trials of its use have been difficult to carry out.

Local anaesthetics

These are most commonly used injected into joints, given intraspinally or, more recently, topically. In a patch format, 5% lignocaine has been used effectively for postherpetic neuralgia. Lignocaine, when given parenterally or in its oral form such as mexilitine, can also be useful for certain types of neuropathic pain (Challapalli et al. 2005).

Bisphosphonates, chemotherapy and radiotherapy

Although these treatments are regularly used where pain is caused by a malignant tumour, or in the case of bisphosphonates to treat osteoporosis, they are mentioned here as they often feature in textbooks for the management of chronic pain. Bisphosphonates can lessen pain in bones by reducing bone reabsorption. Chemotherapy and radiotherapy relieve pain by reducing tumour size, thereby alleviating pressure on local tissues, nerves or organs.

For a useful further text on adjuvant therapy, see Knotkova and Pappagallo (2007).

The role of opioids in the management of non-malignant pain

Before we leave this section, opioids must be considered. Their use in chronic non-malignant pain has been highly controversial, some clinicians believing them to be wholly inappropriate. This view has now changed and a trial of opioids is generally viewed as appropriate for chronic non-malignant pain that is shown to be opioid responsive when other analgesia has failed. Initiating opioids is not without its challenges and a risk/benefit analysis is recommended. The British Pain Society (2005a) offers excellent guidelines for the use of opioids in chronic non-malignant pain. Among the recommendations are:

● The need for a close working relationship between primary and secondary care services about patients who are prescribed opioids.
● The primary outcome should be pain relief, with improvements in physical, psychological and social function as important secondary aims.
● An individualised treatment plan should be developed in discussion with patients.
● Patients should be assessed at regular intervals determined by clinical need.
● The most appropriate way to administer opioids for chronic pain is usually via a long-acting preparation that only needs to be taken once or twice a day, with an immediate-release version of the drug for top-ups or breakthrough pain if needed.

Patch technology now enables patients to apply an opioid patch that only needs to be changed every three days. Some patients are also obtaining relief from opioids, and other drugs, delivered directly to the spine via an implanted **intrathecal** technique. More information about implantable intrathecal drug delivery is available from the British Pain Society (2007).

Regional nerve blocks

In addition to the previous pharmacological interventions, there are a range of special procedures that can be performed, usually by a trained physician, to interrupt the nerve pathways using a wide range of local anaesthetics or nerve ablation techniques.

This is a specialised and extensive field of pain management and therefore will not be covered in any depth here. Further information can be found in some of the many useful textbooks available on this subject, such as Jankovic (2004) or Gymrek and Dahdah (2007).

It is important not to neglect the role of the nurse during these procedures. Recently nurses and other healthcare professionals other than doctors have been acquiring the training and skills to perform nerve blocks; however, nurses' prime responsibility continues to be to provide safety, comfort, reassurance, assessment and information.

Case history

Mrs Brown has had type 1 diabetes for the past 30 years that is controlled by insulin and diet. However, more recently, her glucose control has not been good and her weight has continued to increase steadily over the years. She has been experiencing burning in her feet, especially at night, which stops her sleeping. It was so awful last week that she frequently ran a bath of cold water and sat crying on the edge of the bath, with her feet dangling in the cool water. This brought some relief and she finally went back to bed and slept for short periods. The pain is less in the day but occasionally she gets sharp 'electric shocks' of pain in her feet and numbness especially in her toes.

This type of neuropathic pain is known as 'peripheral diabetic neuropathy'. Successful management of this prevalent condition is reliant upon it being accurately detected and early treatment initiated in primary care. When pain fails to respond to a range of treatments, referral to specialist services (diabetic or chronic pain clinic) may be required. Daousi et al. (2004) and Tölle et al. (2006) explain this pain in more detail and also provide thought-provoking data regarding the large number of people who are experiencing it and often have not mentioned it to their GP.

Non-pharmacological strategies for managing chronic pain

The effective management of chronic pain has to incorporate a range of strategies that have a physical and a psychosocial basis. The following non-pharmacological strategies can be helpful in reducing the perception of pain, while assisting the person to live and cope with his or her pain. It is important to discuss the goal of pain treatment with the person concerned. For example, with chronic pain caused by arthritis, it might be unrealistic to have 'no pain' as a goal, but the person may wish to have a pain level that still allows them to take the children to school or take a short walk in the park.

The following sections reflect the diverse and useful range of strategies available to reduce the impact of pain on a person's life, the intention being to widen approaches to managing pain and to provide you with an opportunity to understand how you might contribute. At this point, however, it must be stressed that nurses should only provide therapies for which they have been appropriately trained, abiding by the NMC code of conduct (2004). Some therapies require basic knowledge. Other strategies, although many still lack regulation, can be practised following the completion of one of the vast range of courses currently available. These courses range from one to two study days in simple massage to a degree course in osteopathy or chiropractic. They are all deemed 'complementary' or 'alternative' approaches, defined as:

> offering diagnosis, treatment and/or prevention that complements mainstream medicine by contributing to a common goal, satisfying a demand not met by orthodoxy or by diversifying the conceptual frameworks of medicine. (Ernst et al. 2001)

In the past, complementary approaches have been slow to gain clinical acceptability because of a lack of rigorous research. Although this is gradually changing, evidence for some of these studies is not compelling. Some cognitive and behavioural therapies have been tested scientifically and have shown clear beneficial effects, but for the most part, it appears that much of the existing research is inconclusive because of common methodological problems with the primary studies (Carroll and Seers 1998). Conducting rigorous trials, for example by performing a sham acupuncture treatment, can be logistically difficult. Also many people who choose complementary therapies believe strongly in their utility and are unwilling to participate in being randomised.

In practice, many people derive benefit, which is not always measurable, from complementary approaches. Relief from pain may not always be the patient's goal: well-being and improved sleep may be other important outcomes and this data is not always collected. As we are now in a climate of evidence-based practice and clinical governance, there is a need not only to be aware of current research, but also to conduct large randomised controlled trials, however difficult these may be in practice. While strong evidence is still lacking, nurses need to be supportive of patients' choices, and they may need to advise and educate about the most appropriate ways to integrate therapies to achieve the best results. The following represent some of the most popular treatments for chronic pain.

Physical techniques for managing pain

Physical strategies using a 'mind–body approach' for managing pain are thought to work by influencing the 'gate control' within the spinal cord and brain, increasing A beta nerve stimulation and in some cases encouraging the release of **endorphins** – the body's own opioids. Some of these techniques are also thought to reduce pain perception by increasing feelings of relaxation and well-being. Many therapists are also in a position to spend more time with patients and this personal interaction may also be beneficial.

Acupuncture

Acupuncture has been practised for thousands of years. Although still not fully understood, it is gaining credibility in Western medicine as a valid treatment for certain types of pain. The technique involves placing fine solid needles into the skin at acupoints along energy pathways termed 'meridians', which are described in classical Chinese medicine.

There is evidence that acupuncture needles stimulate sensory nerves in the skin and muscles, and that these signal to the spinal cord and midbrain. This type of stimulation possibly results in pain modulation via the release of endorphins as well as increasing the discharge of **serotonin** and **noradrenaline** into the central nervous system. It is also thought that the use of acupuncture may work by constricting or dilating blood vessels due to the release of vasodilators such as histamine, but the debate goes on as to just how effective acupuncture is and for what particular conditions (Moore and McQuay 2005). Acupuncture should always be conducted by those trained in its art, as a range of adverse effects, such as pneumothorax and infection, have been associated with its use.

Acupressure

Acupressure is reputed to be even older than acupuncture, although it is not as widely practised. Acupressure is said to produce much the same effect as acupuncture but does not involve needles. Finger or hand pressure is used over the acupoints, which feature along the same energy pathways that form the basis of acupuncture. One form of acupressure is the use of 'sea bands' to treat seasickness. These are elasticated bands, usually about 3cm wide, that have a small, hard button attached to the inside and are worn on the wrist. Researchers have also reported the benefits of using acupressure to treat postoperative nausea and vomiting and for pain relief during transportation to hospital with minor trauma (Kober et al. 2002; Streitberger et al. 2006; Lang et al. 2007). However, there appears to be little in the way of research on its place in chronic pain.

Massage

Massage has certainly been useful in acute pain and would, therefore, probably be beneficial for chronic pain sufferers. It is thought to provide pain relief in a variety of ways. The stimulation of the skin may increase the circulation, which contributes to reduce swelling and promote healing. Touch and massage can stimulate the large diameter A beta fibres, which close the pain gate. The personal attention and relaxation associated with massage can generate a feeling of well-being and modify pain perception. For acute pain, many sportspeople who sustain a painful injury find that their muscles and any damaged tissue respond quickly to moderately deep massage, and they are able to return to the sports field more rapidly. Babies especially have been seen to obtain relief from the pain of colic using gentle massage. Research is beginning to indicate the benefits of massage for patients with a wide range of chronic conditions; for a review, see Tsao (2007).

Physical manipulation

Spinal manipulation particularly is a popular form of treatment for chronic pain and is usually carried out by chiropractors, osteopaths and physiotherapists to treat a range of primarily musculoskeletal problems. The essential characteristic of these therapies is a low or high velocity thrust carefully administered at the end of the normal passive range of movements to increase the joint's range of movement. Like so many treatments, although analysis of multiple studies establishes benefit, there is little evidence that this is superior to effective conventional treatments such as physical therapy, massage, exercise and drug treatments. However, having time with a professional therapist, a usually thorough physical examination, an explanation of why pain is a problem and then the offending areas physically moved beyond their 'comfort zone' can do much to motivate and restore confidence in patients' ability to become more physical. Two reviews for back pain are available from Cherkin et al. (2003) and Assendelft et al. (2003).

Transcutaneous electrical nerve stimulation

Transcutaneous electrical nerve stimulation (TENS) devices were briefly described in Chapter 4; they are thought to work by sending a weak electrical current through the skin to stimulate the sensory nerve endings. This feels like a prickly, buzzing sensation but should not be unpleasant. It is also thought that TENS may help to close the 'gate' in the thalamus of the brain, where pain nerve endings and ordinary touch sensation converge before their final distribution to the cortex of the brain. Some research also suggests that TENS may stimulate the release of endorphins within the brain and spinal cord. TENS may work for all sorts of pain but is usually described as helpful in relieving rheumatic-type aching in joints and muscles, low back pain, amputation stump pain and neuralgia.

Many companies lease TENS machines, along with simple instructions (for example for labour pain and the muscle and joint pain associated with arthritis), to patients, or they can often be purchased in health shops. They are popular because they have no side effects, and some patients derive considerable relief from their pain. Nurses need to know how they work so that they can teach their patients to use the machines safely and confidently.

Despite their widespread use, a review of research in 2000 failed to establish the analgesic effectiveness for TENS in chronic pain, finding insufficient extractable data to make meta-analysis possible (Carroll et al. 2000). New trials of better design are needed; however, where patients do derive benefit from the system, it would seem prudent to continue using it.

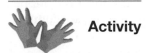

Activity

Find out where you might obtain a TENS machine in your hospital and/or community (they are often available in pharmacies). Identify what you would need to learn in order to recommend its use to a patient or friend and teach them how to use it. Speak to someone who has used a machine and find out how they use it for pain relief – try it yourself too! In many hospitals, physiotherapists are a good source of expertise.

Spinal cord stimulation

Spinal cord stimulation is sometimes used to treat chronic pain that has failed to respond to all other non-invasive therapies. Like TENS, its action is based on the gate control theory of pain. Surgically implanted electrodes, usually placed over the dorsal columns, produce an electrical field to activate pain-inhibiting mechanisms. Not all pain will respond to this kind of treatment but, for carefully selected patients, spinal cord stimulation can provide pain relief. More information is available from the British Pain Society (2005b).

Heat therapy

We all know how good soaking in a warm bath can be: heating the tissues of the body can be very comforting. Warmth to the skin may be another way of closing the gate mechanism in the spinal cord. The conscious feeling of warmth tends to suppress the awareness of pain and helps to promote mental and physical relaxation.

Raising the temperature of damaged tissue may speed up the metabolic process, improve circulation by vasodilatation, reduce oedema and accelerate repair. The heat of a warm bath before activity can reduce the viscosity of synovial fluid, which can reduce painful stiffness in joints with diseases such as arthritis. Starting the day with a warm bath may enable sufferers to function more comfortably. Although we lack research, heat appears to be useful for backache, rheumatic conditions and pain arising from scar tissue or adhesions. Interestingly, when heat is used to treat stomach ache, it can reduce acidity within five minutes. Heat should, however, never be used immediately following tissue damage, as it will increase swelling.

Cold therapy

Cold therapy may also be a way of stimulating nerves to bring about pain modulation, although its value in chronic pain is probably limited and usually unpopular (Carlson 2007). Cold can be applied to treat pain in the form of wrapped crushed ice, and gel-filled cold packs, which are kept in the freezer, are commercially available.

Aromatherapy

Aromatherapy involves the use of essential oils distilled from plants. In addition to having wonderful fragrances, they are also claimed to have specific therapeutic properties that work on the limbic system to reduce tension and stress. They can be used to promote sleep (lavender) and relieve pain (such as clove oil in dentistry). Certain oils, such as tea tree oil, are known to possess an antibacterial action. The oils can be administered in a number of ways: massaged into the skin, dropped neat onto a handkerchief or pillow, used as room sprays, evaporated in special burners, placed in compresses or added to bath water. Again, although we lack rigorous scientific evidence of benefit, so many patients enjoy the experience that it is argued that anecdotal evidence should be sufficient (Howarth 2005). Aromatherapy is available in some areas on the NHS.

Reflexology

Reflexology, like acupuncture, represents a revival of an ancient practice. The therapy is based on the idea that every part of the body has a reflex point on the foot and hand. Therapists use their fingers and hands to produce simple, safe pressure. When an area of tenderness is found, the therapist concentrates on that area by applying pressure in a specific manner to either stimulate or sedate the reflex. It is claimed that the therapy can bring pain relief by 'normalising' organ function and may be useful for dysmenorrhoea, constipation, IBS, urinary retention and premenstrual symptoms.

Psychological interventions

Cognitive behavioural therapy

Cognitive behavioural therapy (CBT) and operant behavioural therapy focus on factors that cause or maintain suffering in chronic pain. As it is generally accepted that behavioural responses to illness and pain are influenced by both positive and negative reinforcements, the therapy works by trying to reinforce the beneficial influences that can improve pain management and encourage positive coping strategies. There is evidence of benefit and it can be argued that these forms of therapy should be routinely considered as part of multidisciplinary treatment (Molton 2007).

Relaxation

Relaxation strategies can utilise a range of interventions. Progressive relaxation is easy to learn and effective. Usually starting at the feet and working up, muscle groups are selected and purposefully tensed for several seconds before being relaxed. Anxiety and muscle relaxation produce the opposite physiological states and therefore cannot exist together.

Seers (1997) describes the impact of a community-based programme using relaxation skills for sufferers of chronic pain. The findings revealed that those patients taught relaxation skills experienced a decrease in their pain intensity and an improvement in sleep in the short and longer term. Schofield (2002) looked at the impact of snoezelen, a multisensory environment enjoyed in a snoezelen room, which is purported to enhance relaxation, and may be especially useful for individuals with learning difficulties or for children.

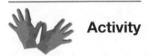 **Activity**

Get into a comfortable position and bring your shoulders up towards your ears. Hold the position for 10 seconds. Then slowly let your shoulders down as low as you possibly can – keep going! What do you notice about your shoulders now? Were you aware of the muscle tensions before you did this exercise?

Biofeedback

Biofeedback is a form of training where patients with chronic pain learn a variety of self-regulation and relaxation strategies to control physiology. Using feedback, patients can learn to reduce muscle tension and muscle guarding. They learn to correct posture and even control autonomic nervous system activity, particularly from the sympathetic nervous system, which is implicated in the amplification and maintenance of pain and stress. Biofeedback training usually includes learning muscle relaxation, diaphragmatic breathing, heart rate control, guided visual imagery and cognitive restructuring. There is research demonstrating the efficacy of these techniques in the treatment of headaches, musculoskeletal conditions such as chronic fatigue and IBS. A small study using thermal feedback in women with endometriosis revealed an improvement in pain and a reduction in the interference of pain on the quality of life (Hawkins and Hart 2003). Although small, this study adds to a number demonstrating the benefits of this approach.

Hypnosis

Hypnosis is as old as mankind and is reported in ancient Egyptian scripts. It lost popularity in the Middle Ages when it was associated with witchcraft. However, there is now a resurgence of interest, with recent controlled studies, despite some methodological flaws, indicating the efficacy of hypnotherapy for the treatment of chronic pain. A review article of controlled trials indicates that hypnotic analgesia produces significantly greater decreases in pain relative to no treatment and to some non-hypnotic interventions such as medication management, physical therapy and education/advice. However, the effects of self-hypnosis training on chronic pain tend to be similar, on average, to progressive muscle relaxation and autogenic training, both of which often include hypnotic-like suggestions (Jensen and Patterson 2006). Research also supports the idea that hypnosis is a genuine physical state and people are not just deceiving themselves into thinking they are hypnotised. Under hypnosis, susceptible individuals show changes in the left frontal cortex of the brain during functional MRI scanning (Gosline 2004).

Guided imagery

Guided imagery often forms part of biofeedback or relaxation therapy and involves forming a mental picture of reality or fantasy, ideally involving all five senses. It is a technique that is relatively easy to use and can be helpful for the treatment of chronic pain and to assist in distraction for short painful procedures. Like other non-pharmacological strategies for acute pain, it should not take the place of analgesia but complement it. Try to make sure that there will be no interruptions and that the environment is warm. Choosing a subject to explore, through the senses, should be agreed between the patient and nurse – maybe a holiday or an activity the patient enjoys.

The following time out is an example of guided imagery. Imagining the scene, see whether you can visualise the image so clearly that you can take your mind off what is going on around you. Imagery that involves natural experiences – the warmth of the sun or sparkling light on the sea – is good to include. You have to concentrate quite hard, some people finding this easier than others.

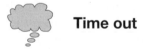 **Time out**

It is a warm summer evening and the wind gently rustles through the leaves on the trees. You are sitting beneath an oak tree and can feel the slightly damp grass beneath you and the warm rays of sun on your skin. In the distance, you hear the sounds of laughter from children playing and the splash of water as they paddle and jump. The fragrant smell of freshly cut grass and heady scent of roses mingle together.

Music therapy

Music therapy can work as a valuable cognitive therapy, with the added benefit that some pieces of music will soothe and relax the listener. Music has been shown to cause the release of endorphins, as well as acting as a cue for relaxation therapy. A personal stereo can be used to listen to music, the volume being increased or decreased in response to the pain; it can even be used at work or while being active. A review of pain and music by Cepeda et al (2004) showed only small benefit but this was conducted on all types of pain. For specific chronically painful conditions such as osteoarthritis pain, music has been shown to be beneficial (McCaffery and Freeman 2003). In studies of patients with chronic pain (Siedliecki and Good 2006), music has also been shown to reduce pain, depression and disability while promoting feelings of power.

Herbs and supplements

Herbal preparations

Herbal medicines are among the most popular forms of complementary treatments, with a large proportion of herbal remedies being used for musculoskeletal pain. Unfortunately, many herbal compounds are developed using 'traditional' knowledge, which is a notoriously unreliable indicator of effectiveness (Ernst et al. 1998). The following are just a selection for which there are some data available:

- Chilli peppers produce capsaicin, now available in a cream (covered briefly in a previous section).
- Devil's claw has been shown to be useful for osteoarthritis pain and low back pain.
- Willow bark, from which aspirin was first developed, has been shown to be useful for low back pain.
- Phytodolor is a mixture of extracts from the flowering plant goldenrod and two tree species, aspen and common ash. It has been shown to be useful for painful arthritic conditions such as rheumatoid arthritis and was reviewed by Bandolier (1997).
- The trees boswellia and winter cherry along with the spices ginger and tumeric have been studied for their anti-inflammatory properties but with mixed results. The last three herbal medicines were reviewed for the treatment of low back pain (Ganier et al. 2007).
- Blackcurrant seeds and borage have so far shown mixed results.
- Evening primrose oil has shown benefit for sufferers of rheumatoid arthritis.

It must be remembered that herbal medicines are not always safe just because they are perceived as 'natural'. Some have quite powerful pharmacologically active ingredients and can interact with a range of medications.

Nutritional supplements

Some nutritional supplements have been shown to be beneficial such as glucosamine, chondroitin and oils from avocado and soya bean for conditions such as osteoarthritis. Omega-3 fatty acids and selenium may be useful for rheumatoid arthritis, while S-adensoyl methionine has been used with some effect for fibromyalgia.

Nurses are often put in a difficult position when asked their opinion about introducing a complementary therapy as they themselves may have little knowledge on the subject. Since it is usually the patient who chooses to use a complementary therapy, they often have a powerful desire for it to be effective. Caution, however, should be advocated in some instances, especially when patients choose herbal preparations as herb/drug and herb/food interactions may occur.

All the above strategies centre on involvement with treatment and exercising a personal sense of control. How individuals perceive their control over a situation will influence how they deal with and respond to it. People with an external locus of control style appear to experience more intense pain than those with an internal locus of control style and this is often coupled with feelings of helplessness, a predictor of higher levels of pain (Hadjistavropoulus and Shymkiw 2007). In chronic pain, treatments that encourage an internal locus of control, such as the self-treatment strategies mentioned above, would appear to have the greatest long-term benefit compared with treatments that are just 'done to' patients.

Other considerations when managing pain

Placebo

It is important to mention the power and, in some cases, the utility of the placebo response. Most people look on placebo as a form of 'mock' medicine. In some instances, before ethics featured so highly, placebo was thought to have a place in demonstrating false claims of pain. The word 'placebo' comes from the Latin 'to please', but a more modern explanation of the placebo effect might be:

> The physician's belief in the treatment and the patient's faith in the physician exert a mutually reinforcing effect; the result is a powerful remedy that is almost guaranteed to produce an improvement and sometimes a cure. (Skrabenek and McCormick 1990, p. 13)

In medical circles, placebos have traditionally been viewed with suspicion, even regarded by some as a nuisance variable in research and by others as an indication of medical charlatanism and quackery (Wall 1992). However, there is now compelling evidence from the literature that placebo analgesia can provoke a powerful response. With the help of brain imaging tools such as positron emission tomography (PET) and functional magnetic resonance imaging (fMRI), our understanding of the role of placebo analgesia has been greatly enhanced (Kong et al. 2007). It is beyond the remit of this book to go into this fascinating subject in more detail and readers are directed to the wide range of literature currently available such as Brody and Brody (2001) and Kradin (2008).

Exercise

For patients suffering chronic pain, establishing a programme of structured physical exercise should be incorporated into strategies to control pain. Although it might at first prove difficult, exercise is thought to be beneficial for the following reasons:

- increases mobility
- enables social interaction
- decreases muscle strain and reduces muscle spasm
- stimulates natural endorphins
- produces stimuli that compete with pain, thereby reducing the perception of pain
- reduces fatigue by increasing stamina
- maintains cardiovascular fitness
- reduces bone demineralisation.

Trusting therapeutic relationships

Creating a trusting nurse–patient relationship is often ignored as a therapeutic intervention. The nursing partnership has been viewed as a way of looking at what happens when the nurse offers expertise to a person who is experiencing a health-related problem (Christensen 1993). This partnership can be an essential component in the management of pain. The ability to convey trust and empathy is a skilled nursing action that requires a partnership in care in which patients and their families are central. Someone experiencing pain is especially vulnerable, and the nurse can be instrumental in helping him or her, not only to cope with the pain, but also to develop some vital skills to communicate when dealing with other healthcare professionals.

Time out

Reflect on the notes you made earlier in this chapter following your interviews with people experiencing chronic pain. Did you notice anything about the 'effect' of taking time to talk with them about their pain? What do you think you were conveying to the patients when you chatted with them, and how might this influence their pain experience?

Living with pain day and night and feeling isolated, depressed and frightened is devastating. This may be compounded if no physical cause can be found for the pain and an endless round of hospital appointments have left the sufferer feeling that no one believes them. Having others believe the pain has been found to be crucial for non-malignant chronic pain sufferers (Seers and Friedli 1996). By discussing pain with your patient, it is likely that you conveyed belief in their pain as well as trust and empathy. This activity of talking openly about pain can ultimately prove highly beneficial in helping patients to cope with what may prove to be an incurable condition.

Social activities

With chronic non-malignant pain, sufferers often become isolated and depressed as a result of the relentless pain they experience. This vicious circle of pain, isolation and depression only causes them to withdraw further, and they often no longer participate in the social activities they once enjoyed so much. Facilitating them to engage in social interaction is important. Meeting friends will help to take their mind off the pain as well as increasing their self-esteem. When pharmacological strategies and medical intervention fail to bring any relief, supporting patients to return to as normal a lifestyle as possible is sometimes the most realistic goal.

Over a period of time, certain patients with pain of unknown aetiology will go on to develop pain behaviours and negative coping strategies, and will adopt the 'sick role'. This results in their withdrawing further from their environment; it alters their role in society so that they become less active, participate less and become totally centred on their own pain. Their management can become very challenging indeed. Chapter 7 will cover some of the issues surrounding the care for patients who fall into this more 'challenging' category.

 Time out

Reflect back on your conversations with your patients. Did they talk about their social life at all? Did they still participate in social events or visits to friends? If they had stopped, why was this? How could they start some of these again?

Professional collaboration in pain management

A variety of professionals can make an important contribution to providing effective pain relief, both as individuals and as part of a specialist team. In the previous section, a range of interventions were identified for the management of pain along with clinicians who may initiate these interventions such as physicians, psychologist, physiotherapists, chiropractors, osteopaths, pharmacists, occupational therapists and specialist nurses, all of whom may be consulted for their expertise and contribution.

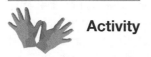 **Activity**

Consider the healthcare professionals in your clinical area who have a role in the management of chronic pain. Make short notes on each of their roles. Now interview each on how they perceive their role in the management of chronic pain.

Are there any other healthcare professionals in your hospital or community who have an interest in pain? How do you access their input? How could you improve collaboration between the many professions with an interest or role in pain management?

It can be quite surprising to discover how many different healthcare professionals have an input into or interest in pain management. All may have their own expertise and approach. When this is communicated effectively and these professionals work together, the impact can be immense. The following section considers how multiprofessional teamwork has made a difference in chronic pain.

Chronic pain clinics

John Lloyd and Samuel Lipton, two enthusiastic anaesthetists, initially proposed the concept of the chronic pain clinic in the 1960s. The techniques originally used were nerve blocks and pharmacological intervention, but clinics now utilise a range of strategies from acupuncture and exercise to biofeedback and psychotherapy, involving a range of professionals. These multidisciplinary pain clinics have become increasingly popular and have adopted a variety of formats. Such clinics often run pain management programmes (PMP), which may be outpatient or inpatient based. Patients may be referred to a chronic pain clinic by their general practitioner or a consultant who has been managing their care. The clinics vary greatly in their structure and management.

The provision of chronic pain services in the UK is increasingly being scrutinised, as the current format of expensive services for a minority of people makes neither moral nor fiscal sense (Dr Foster 2004). Seers (1997) emphasises this point in the rationale to provide a community-based service for people suffering with chronic non-malignant pain, using a simple and cheap intervention (relaxation training). Nurses are ideally placed to develop such services to meet the needs of patients.

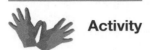 **Activity**

Find out where your nearest chronic pain clinic is situated and identify how patients are referred to it. What facilities does it offer, and how does it evaluate the success of its programmes? Ask for an information sheet about the programme and consider what they focus on. Write this up on a couple of sides of A4 paper.

As previously mentioned, you might discover that such services are few and far between and that interventions might instead continue to focus on pharmacological agents and invasive procedures. Is there a role here for the nurse to develop services utilising some of the non-pharmacological interventions previously discussed in this chapter? Nurse-led services have been developed across a range of patient needs and certainly have scope for considerable input in the management of chronic pain. A nurse may already be involved in the clinic, but in what capacity? Does the role of the nurse actively contribute to helping the patient? Many questions can be asked, but the future looks promising, with a wider recognition of chronic pain. The need to provide care that reaches more people, helping them to improve the quality of their lives, could become a higher priority in the years to come.

Conclusion

When pain does not have a foreseeable end and may have to be endured throughout life, the nurse can help the person and their family to come to terms with this situation and cope with the pain. Educating patients and their families about pain, and drawing on their coping skills, gives the person some control over their life.

This chapter has focused on collecting data from clinical practice to help you to explore how chronic pain is currently being managed in your area. It has given you a framework against which your own experiences and environment can be compared. It is anticipated that this will provide you with the enthusiasm and knowledge to analyse the current management of chronic pain in your practice area and identify methods of influencing change.

After a break, try the multiple choice test below in order to self-assess your understanding so far. For some of the questions, more than one answer will be correct, however, there will be one answer that is so far best supported by the evidence.

Suggested further reading

Allcock N., Elkan R. and Williams J. (2007) Patients referred to a pain management clinic: beliefs, expectations and priorities. *Journal of Advanced Nursing*, **60**(3): 248–56.

Clark D. (2000) Total pain: the work of Ciciely Saunders and the hospice movement. *American Pain Society Bulletin*, **10**(4), http://www.ampainsoc.org/pub/bulletin/jul00/hist1.htm.

Derbyshire S. (2004) Pain and prejudice: our understanding of pain has improved dramatically – so why are we no better at alleviating it?, http://spiked-online.net/Articles/0000000CA50E.htm.

Eliot Cole B. (2007) Advances in opioid analgesia: maximizing benefit while minimizing risk, www.medscape.com/viewprogram/6675. This is quite a complex lecture and is primarily for an American audience but it is an excellent resource for any of you wanting more information about the difficult issue of the assessment of patients with chronic pain who may benefit from opioid analgesia.

Kehlet H., Jensen T. and Woolf C. (2006) Persistent postsurgical pain: risk factors and prevention. *Lancet*, **367**: 1618–25.

McCracken L. and Eccleston C. (2003) Coping or acceptance: what to do about chronic pain? *Pain*, **105**(1/2): 197–204.

Morone N. and Greco C. (2007) Mind-body interventions for chronic pain in older adults: a structured review. *Pain Medicine*, **8**(4): 359–75.

Turk D., Dworkin R, Allen R, Bellamy N, Brandenburg N. et al. (2003) Core outcome domains for chronic pain clinical trials: IMMPACT recommendations. *Pain*, **106**(3): 337–45.

Managing Chronic Pain
Multiple choice TEST

1. What is the principal mode of action of antidepressant drugs when used to treat chronic pain?
   a. They make you feel less depressed so the pain has less of an impact ☐
   b. They make you sleepy so you are more relaxed and less tense ☐
   c. They act centrally to increase the levels of noradrenaline and seratonin ☐
   d. They block the synthesis of bradykinin ☐

2. Why should the assessment and management of pain be documented?
   a. It allows the effectiveness of interventions to be evaluated ☐
   b. It is good practice and professional ☐
   c. It allows other professionals to see how pain is being managed ☐
   d. Documentation formalises the management of pain ☐

3. 'Adjuvant therapy' is the term given to which of the following?
   a. Drugs used to treat the side effects of analgesia ☐
   b. Drugs which aren't analgesics but may provide some pain relief ☐
   c. Drugs used to reverse opioid overdose ☐
   d. Drugs used to treat anxiety and depression ☐

4. Which drug is frequently used as a treatment for chronic pain experienced by patients with or without any obvious pathology?
   a. Steroids ☐
   b. Ketamine ☐
   c. Bisphosphonates ☐
   d. Antidepressants ☐

5. How is it suggested that acupuncture works for the management of pain?
    a. By stimulating the meridians ☐
    b. By stimulating motor nerves in the skin ☐
    c. By taking a person's mind off the pain experience ☐
    d. By stimulating the sensory nerves in the skin and stimulating the release of endorphins ☐

6. Which nerve fibres are beneficially stimulated when using TENS?
    a. C fibres ☐
    b. A beta fibres ☐
    c. Motor nerve fibres ☐
    d. A delta fibres ☐

7. Which of the following has been shown to have a specific effect on gastric acidity?
    a. TENS ☐
    b. Aromatherapy ☐
    c. Acupressure ☐
    d. Heat therapy ☐

8. For patients experiencing chronic non-malignant pain or persistent pain, which of the following has consistently been shown to be the most beneficial?
    a. Having others believe their pain ☐
    b. Regular consultations with a doctor ☐
    c. Rest and the avoidance of physical activity ☐
    d. Regular analgesia ☐

9. Which of the following is not thought to be of specific benefit for people undergoing a structured physical exercise programme?
    a. It increases mobility ☐
    b. It reduces fatigue and increases stamina ☐
    c. It maintains cardiovascular fitness ☐
    d. It improves sleep ☐

10. If you were to identify an improvement that could be made in the management of chronic pain in your area, which would be the most important activity for you to undertake first?
    a. Collect information and undertake an audit to identify current practices ☐
    b. Talk with patients and relatives ☐
    c. Read the current literature on the subject and so on ☐
    d. Implement the 'improvement' ☐

Answers

1. c. They act centrally to increase the levels of noradrenaline and seratonin. They may make you less depressed but the dosages are usually much smaller than those used to treat depression so this is not thought to be significant. Also they may well improve the ability to go to sleep because they cause sedation but the quality of this sleep is sometimes questioned. They are not thought to exert any action on bradykinin.

2. a. It allows the effectiveness of interventions to be evaluated; the documentation of pain assessment and management allows us to share the effectiveness of the selected interven-

tions. Without this record, the patient's response to these interventions cannot be evaluated. This renders interventions ad hoc, resulting in pain management that is often ineffective. It should be noted that all the other answers are also important, although less so.

3. b. Drugs that are not regarded as analgesics but can help to relieve pain by their mode of action. Many of the adjuvant therapies will result in enhanced analgesia when used with traditional analgesic drugs, or on their own to treat specific conditions. For chronic pain, the most frequently used adjuvants are antidepressants and anticonvulsants but there are many others as well.

4. d. Antidepressants; particularly amitriptyline. Steroids are used for inflammatory conditions. Ketamine is an anaesthetic induction agent that is an NMDA receptor antagonist, NMDA being thought to be responsible for the 'wind-up' phenomenon of pain. Bisphosphonates are used to treat the pain arising from bone reabsorbtion that occurs with osteoporosis and certain tumours.

5. d. By stimulating the sensory nerves in the skin, which causes the body to release endorphins; it is thought that this process can result in impulses being transmitted to the brain via the spinal cord and midbrain, causing a modulation response. As a result, the body is stimulated to release its own analgesics – endorphins.

6. b. A beta fibres, the touch and vibration sensation fibres. They conduct the impulses faster than other nerve fibres, and it is thought that the activity generated by this inhibits the activity of the pain nerve fibres within the spinal cord.

7. d. Heat therapy; heat therapy has been shown to reduce gastric acidity within five minutes. There is no data to support a similar response following aromatherapy, acupressure or TENS.

8. a. Having others believe their pain has been shown to be the most important factor in the majority of research so far. Patients may feel that other people do not believe their pain, especially if a cause cannot be found. Answer b may be important for patients with a specific medical condition, but for most patients with chronic pain, the goal would be to not 'medicalise' their pain further when all medical interventions so far have failed. Rest and the avoidance of physical activity are to be discouraged and for sufferers of chronic pain, regular analgesia is rarely effective in the long term.

9. d. It improves sleep; although this may well be the case, research does not support this as being significant for the majority of people, although all the other factors have been identified as being of specific benefit.

10. a. Collect information and audit to identify current practices; this baseline information will be invaluable in establishing what is currently happening so that when you have introduced your 'improvement' (for example a relaxation strategy), you will be able to collect more data and establish whether the improvement in fact made a difference in practice. The process of collecting information will facilitate getting your colleagues involved in being part of the change. Answers b and c described activities in which you could engage when collecting the information. Making a change or implementing an 'improvement' without a, b or c is a recipe for failure.

CHAPTER 6

Managing Pain in Vulnerable Patients

Learning outcomes

On completion of this chapter, the student will be able to:

- Discuss patient groups that are particularly vulnerable to inadequate pain recognition, assessment and management
- Identify a pain assessment strategy for a vulnerable patient and discuss the rationale for the choice
- Analyse factors that might contribute to the inadequate management of pain for these patient groups
- Evaluate strategies that might lead to improved pain relief

Indicative reading

Older people

Brown D. (2004) A literature review exploring how healthcare professionals contribute to the assessment and control of postoperative pain in older people. *International Journal of Older People Nursing/Journal of Clinical Nursing*, **13**(6b): 74–90.

City of Hope, Beckman Research Institute, Special populations, Pain in the elderly, http://prc.coh.org/elderly.asp.

Gibson S. (2006) Older people's pain. *Pain: Clinical Updates*, **14**(3), Seattle, IASP Press, http://www.iasp-pain.org.

Picker Institute (2007) *A Hidden Problem: Pain in Older People*. Oxford, Picker Institute, http://www.pickereurope.org/Filestore/Publications/paincarehomes_final.pdf.

Royal College of Physicians/British Geriatrics Society/British Pain Society (2007) *The Assessment of Pain in Older People: National Guidelines*. Concise Guidance to Good Practice Series, No 8. London, RCP.

Learning disability and brain-injured patients

Kerr D., Cunningham C. and Wilkinson H. (2006) *Responding to the Pain Experiences of People with a Learning Difficulty and Dementia*. University of Edinburgh, Joseph Rowntree Foundation, http://www.jrf.org.uk/bookshop/eBooks/9781859354599.pdf.

Lewis S., Bell D. and Gillanders D. (2007) Managing chronic pain in people with learning disabilities: a case study. *British Journal of Learning Disabilities*, **35**: 93–8.

Pollard M. (2007) Is it pain: a framework for identifying pain in people with learning disabilities. *Practice and Research*, **10**(6): 12–14.

Neonates and preverbal children

Anand K. and the International Evidence-based Group for Neonatal Pain (2001) Consensus statement for the prevention and management of pain in the newborn. *Archives of Pediatrics & Adolescent Medicine*, **155**: 173–80.

Duhn L. and Medves J. (2004) A systematic integrative review of infant pain assessment tools. Advances in Neonatal Care, *Medscape*, http://www.medscape.com/viewarticle/484129.

Cignacco E., Hamers J., Stoffel L., van Lingen R., Gessler P. et al. (2007) The efficacy of non-pharmacological interventions in the management of procedural pain in preterm and term neonates: a systematic literature review. *European Journal of Pain*, **11**: 139–52.

RCN (Royal College of Nursing) (2000) Clinical practice guidelines: the recognition and assessment of acute pain in children: Technical report, http://www.rcn.org.uk/development/practice/clinicalguidelines/pain.

Ethnic minorities

Davidhizar R. and Giger J. (2004) A review of the literature on care of clients in pain who are culturally diverse. *International Nursing Review*, **51**: 47–5.

Background

Until recently, if you were to look through the literature on the assessment and management of pain, the vast majority of it explored pain experienced by patients able to communicate verbally. Being able to communicate effectively makes the assessment and treatment of pain relatively straightforward: you and your patient can join together as a team to experiment with interventions and evaluate their efficacy using a variety of well-tested assessment tools. For some patients, however, the ability to communicate may be absent, impaired or not yet developed. Alternatively, cultural and language differences may hamper adequate assessment and treatment as well as the resignation and stoicism often associated with older populations. Although much of the work on assessment remains experimental and needs further development, in the past few years we have seen some useful tools and clinical guidelines appearing that can assist in managing pain in vulnerable groups of patients. Drawing on our own experiences and contemporary literature, we have assembled some of the key points for providing pain relief for vulnerable groups. We would like to stress, however, that the challenges in applying some of our newly acquired knowledge to the more vulnerable cannot be underestimated. Although things have improved in the management of pain in prever-bal infants and children, for older persons, particularly with cognitive impairment, it would appear that the situation is very slow to improve (Fries et al. 2001; Higgins et al. 2004; Hester 2007; Picker Institute 2007).

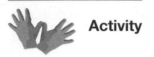 **Activity**

Carry out a brief literature search to identify articles on pain management in a particularly vulnerable client group. Do you notice any gaps or difficulties? Why do you think this might be?

'Vulnerable' is often defined as 'capable of being physically or emotionally wounded or hurt', and a computer thesaurus listed alternative descriptions such as 'defenceless, exposed, susceptible, unprotected and weak'. An editorial in *Nursing Clinics of North America* begins by stating:

> Vulnerable populations are social groups who experience relatively more illness, premature death, and diminished quality of life than comparable groups. Vulner-able populations are often poor; many are discriminated against or subordinated; and they are frequently marginalized and disenfranchised. Vulnerable populations typically include women and children, ethnic people of colour, immigrants, the homeless, the elderly, and gay men and women. (Flaskerud 1999, pp. xv–xvi)

In particular, we shall be looking at how communication difficulties are the prin-cipal factors that render these patients vulnerable or susceptible to hurt through the inadequate recognition and treatment of their pain.

You will probably find that the more vulnerable your patient group, the less has been written or researched on the subject of their pain management. In fact, Liebes-kind and Melzack (1987) said that 'pain is most poorly managed in those who are most defenceless against it'. This is probably because it is particularly difficult not only to assess this group of patients, but also to find and evaluate a therapy that will provide the optimum response for the least side effects.

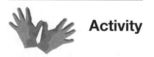 **Activity**

Skim the index and some of the chapters of a pain textbook to see whether atten-tion is paid to vulnerable people. What do you notice? If pain management is mentioned in this context, do the books stress the 'difficulty', or do they give practical help on how to manage or approach specific problems?

Vulnerable patients can baffle us with the complexity of their needs, but providing adequate analgesia is not impossible, as we shall see later from some case histories. Before we go any further, it might be useful to define some of the vulnerable patient groups that this chapter will discuss. We should stress that the list of groups identified is not exhaustive, but we aim to cover a wide selection of people. We start by looking at the needs of the older person, and then move on to those particularly suffering with cognitive impairment, whether their state has arisen as the result of age-related Alzheimer's disease or senile dementia. The next section covers patients with severe learning disabilities and those who, following a stoke or trauma, suffer from brain damage. We shall also be looking at the needs of neonates and preverbal children, and the associated communication problems. Lastly, we briefly consider some of the work that has been done with patients from different ethnic backgrounds, who may encounter language problems, who may be unable to convey their thoughts and feelings to staff from a different culture, or for whom pain has a meaning different from our own.

These are, of course, not the only groups of patient who have traditionally experienced inadequate pain management as a result of communication problems, misconception, knowledge deficit or even prejudice. Chapter 7 will investigate the pain management needs of patients whose pain is complex and challenging; those with psychosocial or behavioural problems, complex pathologies or a history of substance abuse.

Defining the barriers

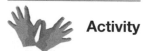 **Activity**

List the patients whom you can think of who have suffered inadequate pain assessment/management. What do you consider were the difficulties of pain management for each of them? When you have collected the information, try to summarise your findings. Putting the answers into a table format can be helpful, with the vulnerable groups listed across the top and potential problems such as communication or compliance problems, knowledge deficit, non-existent assessment, institutional barriers and so on listed down the side. This may help you to categorise the various problems encountered by each client group.

Having carried out this exercise, you may now be clearer in your own mind as to what particular difficulties your patient groups may experience. Once we are aware of the problems we face, we are then in a better position to devise solutions.

Pain in the older person

There is now a major shift in the age distribution of the world's population, with the percentage of 65-year-olds and above expected to reach over 35% in developed countries by 2050 and the number of over 80-year-olds set to triple (US Bureau of the Census 2004). Evidence strongly suggests that pain and cognitive impairment may coexist in a high proportion of older persons. As Parmelee (1996) states: 'the management of either problem alone is a challenge; their concurrence may well test the limits of the skills of professional and informal caregivers alike'. With an increasingly older population, it is essential that we develop the knowledge and skills to manage pain in this group of people effectively.

In studies from nursing homes around the developed world, the incidence of pain has been reported to be as high as 80% (Higgins et al. 2004). Marzinski (1991) reported that 70% of nursing home residents indicated that they had pain and 34% had constant pain, while 66% reported intermittent pain. Despite the prevalence of pain, only 15% of the patients had received any analgesia in the previous 24 hours. Although more recent studies have shown an increasing use of analgesia (Picker Institute 2007), its selection and evaluation appears to be inconsistent and haphazard, with a small proportion of nursing home residents still reporting untreated 'excruciating' daily pain.

One of the first problems to tackle is that of pain assessment. Go into any areas that deal with the care of the older person, whether or not cognitively impaired, and, given the extent of the problem, doesn't it strike you as odd that pulse, blood pressure and bowel movement may be recorded periodically but it is doubtful that you will find a similar record of pain assessment and medication evaluation? A recent review of pain in older residents of nursing homes (Picker Institute 2007) came to the following conclusions:

- Chronic pain is widespread, which leads to staff and residents accepting pain as an inevitable consequence of growing old
- The effects of chronic pain reduce quality of life, limit mobility, restrict social life, and cause depression, irritability and tiredness
- The management of pain is heavily dependent on basic analgesia dispensed on a routine rather than an individualised basis
- Medication is often viewed with suspicion and taken reluctantly
- Residents rarely see their GPs and take little part in a medication review
- A high level of stoicism exists
- Staff fail to ask about pain
- There is a failure to explore alternative pain-relieving strategies
- Some equipment such as hoists can exacerbate discomfort
- Activities that can alleviate pain or offer comfort are often dependent on staff time.

Case history

Mr Hopkin is 86 years old and has had a chronic back problem for many years. This was diagnosed five years ago as spinal stenosis and over the years he has managed on paracetamol 1g and ibuprofen 400mg taken as needed. He also has quite advanced heart disease and arthritis in his hips. Over the past couple of months, Mr Hopkin's back pain has got considerably worse and despite taking his usual analgesia, this is insufficient to control his pain and he is becoming increasingly distressed. He goes to his doctor who records Mr Hopkin's pain intensity as 8/10 using a standard numerical assessment tool. Further questioning reveals that Mr Hopkin is experiencing sleep disturbance and is showing signs of depression. His wife died at the beginning of the year and this has hit him quite hard. The GP prescribes oxycodone 5mg with paracetamol 1g four times a day on a regular basis. Applying a NSAID topically rather than taking it orally is also suggested, as Mr Hopkin has advanced heart disease and long-term systemic use of NSAIDs is not recommended. However, this is subsequently discounted as impractical as there is nobody available to give Mr Hopkin assistance in its application. A stimulant laxative to be taken at night is also prescribed to avoid constipation and, with Mr Hopkin's agreement, he is commenced on a selective serotonin and noradrenaline reuptake inhibitor (SSNRI) antidepressant.

Over the next couple of weeks Mr Hopkin's pain as well as his symptoms of constipation, depression and fatigue are assessed by the practice nurse during a regular telephone follow-up assisted by the Brief Pain Inventory and some additional questioning. As a result of these follow-ups, Mr Hopkin needs several adjustments to his medications. He is given a prescription for some immediate-release oxycodone 5mg for breakthrough pain to be taken up to three times a day in addition to his regular analgesia. He is also given advice about increasing his laxatives, drinking more fluids, using a warm pad over his lower back when sitting in a chair and trying to increase his daily activity as his pain control improves.

After six weeks, Mr Hopkin comes back to see his GP about reducing his medications as his pain is now well controlled, he is sleeping much better, his mood has improved and he is even finding he can get into the potting shed again and grow some seedlings for his vegetable patch. He is now much more confident that when his back pain flares up again, there are medications and strategies available to help alleviate the worst of his symptoms.

People with a pain-eliciting pathology may well be very accepting of their discomfort and 'lot in life', and have a low expectation for relief. For patients who can communicate, there is no reason why pain cannot be assessed using the 'gold standard' of self-report and strategies based on this assessment selected to ameliorate their suffering. For those who cannot communicate effectively, it is up to us to ensure that if a painful condition exists, we are aware of it. We then need to be more creative in our approach to the assessment and management of these patients' pain.

Gibson and Helme (1995) pointed out that fewer than 25% of individuals remain disability free by the age of 70 years and fewer than 15% by the age of 80. You may be able to think of a considerable list of conditions associated with ageing that can blight the enjoyment of retirement. Table 6.1 may help to highlight some of the more common potential causes of pain.

Table 6.1 Common causes of pain in the older person

Type of pain	Cause
Musculoskeletal pain	Osteoarthritis, osteoporosis, rheumatoid arthritis, **gout**, **polymyalgia rheumatica**, **giant cell arteritis**, trauma following falls
Malignant pain	The prevalence of cancer increases with age. Tumour growth may lead to nerve compression, pain from **bony metastasis**, raised intracranial pressure, visceral pain and **lymphoedema**. Treatments can lead to nerve damage following radiotherapy; postoperative pain following surgery and medications may lead to constipation or sore mouth
Abdominal pain	Serious intra-abdominal pathology increases with age, for example **biliary disease**, **diverticular disease** and ruptured **aortic aneurysm**. Interestingly, some of the less serious pathologies such as appendicitis may actually decrease in later years
Cardiovascular pain	Angina, intermittent claudication of the legs, **venous leg ulcers**, **post-stroke pain**
Virus infection	**Postherpetic neuralgia**
Diseases	Parkinson's disease and MS. Diabetes, which can lead to painful peripheral neuropathy, tissue damage and ulcers

The approach to the assessment of pain in older people able to communicate is basically the same as for any other adult with a few additional considerations. Pain, depression, loneliness and dementia may feature more frequently as well as some physical disabilities that need to be considered.

These are some simple strategies to improve pain management in the older person:

- Identify any sensory loss such as impaired hearing or vision and ensure patients have glasses on and hearing aids in.
- Communicate clearly sitting close and preferably in front of your patient so they can lip-read if necessary. Avoid standing at the end of the bed and try not to shout.
- Use touch to convey your interest in their pain. It also encourages active listening.
- Explore personal beliefs and potential barriers to effective treatment such as fear of medication side effects. Many older people feel they already take too many drugs and are reluctant to take analgesia even when it proves effective.
- Where possible, include the family or carer in any plans, as patient forgetfulness may hamper attempts to improve pain control.
- Always select an appropriate pain assessment tool that the patient understands and is happy to use. For acute pain, most older people will be happy with a verbal rating scale, although some will prefer to use a numerical rating or faces scale. Less

popular appears to be the visual analogue scale. For chronic pain, any of the recognised validated assessment tools seem to work quite well but will need to be carefully explained.

Pain management in the cognitively impaired older person

There is unfortunately little research examining the ability of healthcare professionals or family members to estimate pain in the cognitively impaired person, although there are some data to indicate that, so far, we have all been doing rather badly. Healthcare professionals appear to be particularly poor at pain estimation, the bulk of the evidence tending to show an underestimation of pain intensity (Weiner et al. 1998; Cohen-Mansfield and Lipson 2002). Dementia or brain injury and its consequent problems, such as impaired formal thinking, lead to the formation of less sophisticated concepts of pain. This may then cause painful pathology to be masked or missed altogether because of behavioural disturbances (Corran and Melita 1998). Perhaps more alarming is the fact that when healthcare professionals do recognise that pain is probably present, they fail to prescribe and administer analgesia as they would for those patients able to communicate (Morrison and Siu 2000).

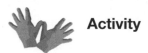 **Activity**

What is it like in your area? What percentage of your older cognitively impaired patients do you think experience regular pain? During one shift, ask each older patient in your clinical area who can communicate verbally whether he or she experiences pain on a regular basis. Given that you were only asking those older patients able to communicate their pain, what percentage overall do you now think experience regular pain?

Now you have ascertained the extent of pain in this population, it is probably safe to estimate that the prevalence of pain is pretty much the same for those unable to express their pain verbally. So far, there is no consistent evidence to indicate that people with dementia experience significantly less pain sensation (Gibson and Farrell 2004), although a complication of pain assessment for older adults with dementia is that their expression of pain sometimes takes on a less obvious form such as confusion, aggression, behavioural changes and social withdrawal (Herr et al. 2006).

Where verbal communication is not possible, nonverbal behaviours should be considered. Nurses need to observe nonverbal cues, such as facial expression and gross motor behaviour. We now have plenty of research on nonverbal expressions of pain in cognitively intact patients of all ages, which tend to show consistency in both facial and 'body language' indicators of pain.

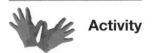
Activity

Choose three cognitively impaired older patients whom you consider could be in pain. These patients could be suffering dementia from a variety of causes, for example Alzheimer's disease. Are you able to identify certain behaviours that you feel may consistently indicate the presence of pain? Are you aware of any potentially painful conditions that each patient may have?

Even for patients with moderate cognitive impairment, it is usually possible to self-report pain using simple, specific questions and maybe a verbal or faces rating scale. When this is not possible, then observable indicators of the potential presence of pain, listed in Table 6.2, have been incorporated into a wide range of assessment tools for the cognitively impaired.

Table 6.2 Observable indicators of the potential presence of pain in cognitively impaired older people

Facial expressions	Slight frown; sad, frightened face Grimacing, wrinkled forehead, closed or tightened eyes Any distorted expression Rapid blinking
Verbalisations, vocalisations	Sighing, moaning, groaning Grunting, chanting, calling out Noisy breathing Asking for help Verbally abusive
Body movements	Rigid, tense body posture, guarding Fidgeting Increased pacing, rocking Restricted movement Gait or mobility changes
Changes in interpersonal interactions	Aggressive, combative, resisting care Decreased social interactions Socially inappropriate, disruptive Withdrawn
Changes in activity patterns and routines	Refusing food, appetite change Increase in rest periods Sleep, rest pattern changes Sudden cessation of common routines Increased wandering
Mental status changes	Cryng or tears Increased confusion Irritability or distress

Source: Reproduced with permission from the American Geriatrics Society (2002) The management of persistent pain in older persons. *Journal of the American Geriatrics Society*, **50**(6): s205–24, http://www. americangeriatrics.org/products/positionpapers/JGS5071.pdf

If you have worked in long-term healthcare settings, or indeed any setting where pain relief is more challenging, you will probably have observed many of these behaviours that appear to be associated with pain. Unfortunately, behaviours aren't necessarily an indication of pain as some patients may demonstrate little or no specific behaviour. The use of facial expression can also be inaccurate for patients who have Parkinson's disease or cerebrovascular damage (Forsyth 2007). Other responses to pain may include physiological changes such as sweating, flushing/blanching of the skin, tachycardia or raised blood pressure. Patients may become agitated, irritable or aggressive with fluctuating cognition. They may become weepy and withdrawn, changing their usual routine and even become more at risk of falls.

 Time out

Having identified some of the behaviours you might observe, how would you measure them? What sort of criteria would you use?

Measurement scales for observation can be devised by using simple categories such as 'none', 'a little' 'quite bad' or 'a lot'. Although these seem quite straightforward, they are not always reliable, as they require the subjective judgement of the observer. One person might judge 'a little' to be the same as another's 'a lot'. To avoid discrepancy between the different assessors, it is helpful to have some sort of quantitative measure, for example none = 0, a little = 1–3, quite bad = 4–7 and a lot = 8–10. A description to verify the score makes the judgement less subject to bias and can be particularly helpful.

Case history

Mrs Bruce is admitted to an orthopaedic ward from a residential care home with a fractured neck of femur. She has a longstanding history of dementia, no close relatives, and there has been little liaison between the nursing home and the orthopaedic ward staff. Prior to her surgery, the nursing home described Mrs Bruce as quiet and withdrawn.

Several hours after returning from theatre following a hip replacement, Mrs Bruce becomes noisy and obviously distressed. She is given an intravenous opioid (morphine 5mg) and settles rapidly. Two hours later, she is once again noisy and distressed. No formal pain assessment has been commenced, the only documentation stating the fact that she received opioid analgesia two hours previously. Her opioid analgesia, now in the form of codeine with paracetamol 1g, is prescribed 4–6-hourly prn, with no additional analgesia for breakthrough pain or regular NSAID should this regime prove inadequate on its own. For the next hour, Mrs Bruce becomes progressively noisier and disturbs the other patients. She is given her codeine/paracetamol but she rapidly becomes agitated again. She is given a seda-tive and eventually quietens down. Over a period of 12 hours, this pattern is repeated, a sedative being administered more regularly than analgesia. A senior nurse then commences an 'observed behaviour pain assessment chart' based on Mrs Bruce's level of restlessness, noise and distress. The nurse also suggests that ibuprofen and paracetamol, without codeine, are given on a regular basis; with oral morphine 5–20mg prescribed hourly prn for breakthrough pain. The change in Mrs Bruce is immediate and positive. After a couple of days, a nurse from the nursing home calls in to see how Mrs Bruce is doing and how she will manage when discharged. She comments that Mrs Bruce has shown a high tolerance to codeine in the past but this was not noted in any of her documentation.

Poor pain management had changed Mrs Bruce from her normally quiet, seemingly content but somewhat withdrawn self to someone showing behaviour that was noisy, disruptive and very distressed. Once adequate pain assessment had been introduced and effective analgesia administered, based on the findings from this assessment, the patient changed back to her usual self. She required no further sedation and went on to regain her previous mobility. Through a rehabilitation programme, she was discharged to her home a week later.

You might think that the above scenario is uncommon and that elderly patients are never left to suffer pain. Unfortunately, however, the evidence suggests that Mrs Bruce's earlier treatment is far from rare. Although now somewhat dated, Wall and Jones (1991) provide a chilling summary of a case that occurred in 1988 in an NHS teaching hospital in which a frail elderly woman in severe pain from a fractured femur was ignored. Her cries disturbed other patients so she was moved to a dark side room with no bell or light switch. This was not necessarily the behaviour of a callous, uncaring nurse. Referral to Chapter 5 highlights the problems associated with the poor prescribing habits of medical staff, the non-existence of pain assessment, misconceptions surrounding the use of powerful analgesia and the bureaucratic barriers that can sometimes leave nurses feeling powerless to remedy a situation in which they only play a part.

How could Mrs Bruce's initial situation have been avoided? Would it have been useful to ask the carers at Mrs Bruce's home about her normal behaviour and previ-ous response to analgesia? They may be able to provide useful information about what a particular behaviour might indicate, whether the patient normally responds to pain or discomfort in this way and what the possible causes of pain may be when they are not as blindingly obvious as a fractured femur. They can also provide infor-mation about what may have been a useful treatment in the past. Using an 'around-the-clock' prescription for analgesia might have avoided some of the problems. Inserting a hip block and being able to top this up with local anaesthetic, although not the norm yet in most hospitals, may have been useful, avoiding the side effects associated with NSAID and opioid analgesia (Layzell 2007). All these strategies will help you to devise a way of assessing and managing pain in the cognitively impaired older person more effectively.

A pain diary or similar documentation that stays with patients and can be taken with them when they change environments could be invaluable. It could be used by staff or relatives to document any pain management strategies that have been successful, or less so, in the past, as well as any adverse effects that the therapy may have produced. Pain in the confused elderly is so often overlooked or dismissed. It would seem that, like neonates, many confused elderly patients have suffered from the assumption that they cannot feel pain, or staff feel concerned about giving them analgesia unnecessarily. This should not be the case. A trial period of analgesia and regular documentation of their pain behaviour is an effective way of assessing analgesic requirements. Remember too that mild pain can respond well to additional strategies, such as comfort, touch, massage, warm baths, heat pads and distraction.

Table 6.3 gives examples of pain assessment tools devised specifically to aid pain management for the nonverbal older adult. None of these tools are perfect but they provide a basis on which to develop some rational strategies to improve care in this particularly vulnerable group.

Table 6.3 Pain assessment tools to aid pain management for the nonverbal older adult

• Abbey Pain Scale (Abbey et al. 2004)
• Assessment of Discomfort in Dementia (ADD) Protocol (Kovach et al. 1999)
• Checklist of Nonverbal Pain Indicators (CNPI) (Feldt 2000)
• Discomfort Scale-Dementia of the Alzheimer's Type (DS-DAT) (Hurley et al. 1992)
• Doloplus 2 (Lefebvre-Chapiro 2001)
• Face, Legs, Activity, Cry and Consolability (FLACC) Pain Assessment Tool (Merkel et al. 1997)
• Nursing Assistant-Administered Instrument to Assess Pain in Demented Individuals (NOPPAIN) (Snow et al. 2004)
• Pain Assessment in Advanced Dementia (PAINAD) Scale (Warden et al. 2003)
• Pain Assessment for the Dementing Elderly (PADE) (Villaneuva et al. 2003)
• Pain Assessment Checklist for Seniors with Limited Ability to Communicate (PACSLAC) (Fuchs-Lacelle and Hadjistavropoulos 2004)

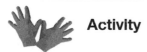 **Activity**

It can be difficult to identify which tool is the most appropriate for your patient. Have a look at the review by Herr et al. (2006) or log on to the website referred to at the end of this section and choose a tool you think will be most helpful. Make some notes on why you chose this tool.

Choosing an assessment tool is a difficult task. A review can be helpful in bringing together a summary of which tool might be the most reliable (repeated measurement of pain gets the same results with different people using it) and valid (it measures what it says it is measuring, for example pain behaviour). Some tools have been created to use in research study and are not particularly easy to use in clinical practice on an everyday basis – they can be time-consuming to complete. Hopefully the tool you chose will be easy to use, can be completed in a timely manner and you found the component questions/observations relevant and helpful.

Examples of useful assessment tools are available from the City of Hope, Beckman Research Institute website, http://prc.coh.org/elderly.asp. In addition, these tools have been the subject of a 'state-of-the-science' review by Herr et al. (2006). Additional assessment tools include pain behaviour measure, proxy pain questionnaire, facial action coding system and facial grimace scale. As you can see, there are plenty to choose from, all of which have been developed in the past decade or so.

The basic principles for good pain management in older people in an ideal world can be summarised as follows:

- Introduce pain assessment for healthcare practitioners and carers with a toolkit and education strategy to go with it.
- Develop simple guidelines on pain and its management for care homes, carers and patients.
- Every case should be treated individually, with treatment adapted to individuals' needs.
- There should be some sort of 'shared record card' to pass information to relevant parties.
- For older people living in the community, carers and family should be trained and supported, ideally with telephone support and an emergency number to call.
- Improve communication between primary, secondary and residential care, with a link person available to provide advice on pain management.
- Routinely assess for other factors associated with pain such as poor sleep pattern and depression.

The above represent key action points suggested by Hester (2007), president of the British Pain Society at the time. Some of these will need concerted organisational change but other, more simple strategies such as selecting and implementing assessment tools and evaluating the effect of analgesia are attainable goals to reach in whichever clinical area you work.

Further reading

American Geriatrics Society (2002) *The Management of Persistent Pain in Older Persons*, http://www.americangeriatrics.org/products/positionpapers/JGS5071.pdf.

Australian Pain Society (2005) *Pain in Residential Aged Care Facilities: Management Strategies*, http://www.apsoc.org.au/owner/files/9e2c2n.pdf.

Cohen-Mansfield J. and Lipton S. (2008) The utility of pain assessment for analgesic use in persons with dementia. *Pain*, 134(1/2): 16–23.

Crome P., Main C. and Lally F. (2007) *Pain in Older People*. Oxford, Oxford University Press.

Herr K., Bjoro K. and Decker S. (2006) Tools for assessment of pain in nonverbal older adults with dementia: a state-of-the-science review. *Journal of Pain and Symptom Management*, 31(2): 170–92.

Herr K., Coyne P., Key T., Manworren R., McCaffery M. et al. (2006) Pain assessment in the nonverbal patient: position statement with clinical practice recommendations. *Medscape*, http://www.medscape.com/viewarticle/533939.

McCleane G. and Smith H. (2006) *Clinical Management of the Elderly Patient in Pain*. Binghamton, NY, Haworth Press.

Ranjan R. (ed.) (1995) *Chronic Pain in Old Age: An Integrated Biospsychosocial Perspective*. Toronto, University of Toronto Press.

Thomas N. (ed.) (1997) *Pain: Its Nature and Management*. London, Baillière Tindall. (Specific chapters deal with the management of children's pain and management strategies for pain in the elderly.)

Walker J., Akinsanya J., Davis B. and Marcer D. (1990) The nursing management of elderly patients with pain in the community: study and recommendations. *Journal of Advanced Nursing*, 15: 1154–61.

Weiner D., Herr K. and Rudy T. (2003) *Persistent Pain in Older Adults: An Interdisciplinary Guide to Treatment*. New York, Springer.

Learning disability and brain-injured patients

The difficulties encountered for patients with any cognitive impairment are similar to those of elderly patients suffering from dementia and evidence suggests that, as for them, pain is often not identified and is therefore undertreated (Kerr et al. 2006). However, the care of brain-injured patients can highlight some added challenges that have to be considered; not least of these is the conclusion that people with learning disabilities are more likely to experience painful conditions than the general population (DH 2001; Stallard et al. 2001). Unfortunately, patients with learning difficulties are sometimes described as being victims of 'diagnostic overshadowing'. This term is used to describe when a change in behaviour is assumed to be part of the learning disability, which then leads to a health problem being missed, sometimes with tragic consequences. In addition, there is a common misconception that people with learning disabilities have a higher tolerance to pain (Folley and McCutcheon 2004). Although some may have impairment to neural pathways and pain insensitivity, others may display a hypersensitivity to pain (Biersdorff 1994). The difficulties associated with their care will depend on their degree of disability and handicap; however, even when able to communicate pain, Kerr et al. (2006) concluded that this was no guarantee that the patient would receive sufficient, if any, pain relief. As with the elderly, various descriptors have been used to guide their care and assessment, although so far there have been few tools devised specifically for this group of patients.

While self-report, however limited, will always be the goal for pain assessment, other methods can be successful, especially when staff and relatives are able to identify patients' unique ways of expressing pain, sometimes in the face of severe disability. With the brain injured and those with severe learning disabilities, the key to successful treatment will hinge on being able to establish what their normal pre-pain behaviour was like and then listing those changes in behaviour that appear to be associated with pain.

Assessment tools have been used with apparent success in the past. These include using a functional analysis as part of a pain assessment test (Astor 2001) or using the

Pain and Discomfort Scale (PADS) (Bodfish et al. 2001). Regnard et al. (2007) describe the development of the Disability Distress Assessment Tool (DisDAT), which has been piloted for patients with severe communication difficulties. There was no evidence from their study that pain had any specific signs or behaviours but assessing distress was a useful clinical guide. For a guide on other assessment tools, either trialed or under development, see the NLH Learning Disabilities Specialist Library (2007). The key is to have a detailed history available that provides information on how a patient has expressed pain in the past and also some sort of record of previous analgesia used and a documented response. The family or a carer who knows the person really well will often detect changes in their behaviour indicative of pain or distress.

Further reading

Harper K. and Bell S. (2006) A pain assessment tool for patients with limited communication ability. *Nursing Standard*, **20**(51): 40–4.
Defrin R., Pick C., Peretz C. and Carmeli E. (2004) A quantitative somatosensory testing of pain threshold in individuals with mental retardation. *Pain*, **108**(1/2): 58–66.
Phan A., Edwards C. and Robinson E. (2005) The assessment of pain and discomfort in individuals with mental retardation. *Research in Developmental Disabilities*, **26**(5): 433–9.
Zwakhalen S., van Dongen K., Hamers J. and Abu-Sd H. (2004) Pain assessment in intellectually disabled people: non-verbal indicators. *Journal of Advanced Nursing*, **45**(3): 236–45.

Neonates and preverbal children

Not only do neonates lack the ability to communicate, small children also experience communication problems. As a group, their pain management needs have probably, until recently, been the most neglected of all. It is only during the past decade or so that our ignorance and widespread misconceptions about neonatal and early childhood neurological development have been challenged. For years, it was felt that neonates and infants did not feel pain as their neuroanatomy and neurochemistry were immature. As recently as the early 1980s, cardiac surgery was described where no analgesia was administered at all. Research now indicates that the reverse may well be the case, that because of the immaturity of pain-modulating systems, neonates may actually experience more pain than adults. Contrary to previous thinking, we now know that neonates exhibit behavioural, physiological and hormonal responses to pain (Fitzgerald 1993). There is also accumulating evidence to suggest that neonates have pain perception beginning in the second trimester (Anand and Maze 2001), with the development of the endorphin and inhibitory systems in the descending pain pathways not completely functional until term, making preterm infants potentially more sensitive to pain than term infants (Anand and Scalzo 2000). We still have a way to go before we fully understand the impact of pain in the neonate, but there are suggestions that repetitive and prolonged pain exposure may permanently modify the developing nervous system. This may manifest itself in lowered pain thresholds during later infancy (Ruda et al. 2000; Bhutta et al. 2001), hypoalge-sia (a diminished sensation of pain) after puberty but hyperalgesia (extreme sensitivity to pain) in adulthood (Ren et al. 2004).

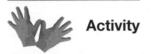 **Activity**

Ask three colleagues what they consider to be the difficulties associated with pain management for neonates and preverbal small children.

These difficulties will be faced by all units dealing with this vulnerable group of patients, so it may be useful to look around and see how other people have responded. Good practice is so often shared only via journal articles or during conferences and is not, therefore, readily available or adequately disseminated to ward staff. The appointment of a link nurse, or utilising the expertise of staff on specialist courses, is often overlooked or undervalued. Developing a journal group to peruse the relevant literature and obtain copies for other staff members to read is also a good way of passing on good practice.

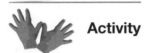 **Activity**

Which assessment tools have you seen used in your clinical area? Are these tools easy to understand and use. Do you think these tools work well? Jot down some notes about what makes an assessment tool user friendly and applicable to clinical practice rather than research.

Many groups are now studying different aspects of neonatal and infant behaviour in order to assess pain, concentrating on facial expressions, body movements and crying. In some cases, physiological indicators of pain such as heart rate, respiratory rate, blood pressure, oxygen saturation (SaO_2), **vagal tone**, palmar sweating, plasma **cortisol** or **catecholamine** levels have been recorded as measures of distress. Although currently time-consuming and somewhat unwieldy, these assessments show promise. Striving for valid assessment tools is vital if we are to combat the stress response to pain in the neonate and the deleterious effect that this may have on their recovery. So far there are conceptual and measurement issues with pain assessment and no specific measure has been set as a gold standard (Cignacca et al. 2007). In addition, different pain assessment tools may work in different circumstances for different reasons, and practitioners may need to adapt and individualise an assessment tool as necessary depending on clinical circumstances (Duhn and Medves 2004).

There are currently more than 40 pain assessment tools available and most of these have been developed to measure acute procedural or short-term pain and only three have been developed for more prolonged pain (Ranger et al. 2007). Table 6.4 provides a list of some assessment tools but readers are directed to Duhn and Medves (2004) for a systematic review of infant pain assessment tools and the Royal College of Nursing's clinical practice guidelines (RCN 2000). Whichever tool is selected, it is important to ensure that all staff use exactly the same criteria to measure pain and distress. Some of the assessment tools in Table 6.4 can be downloaded from the internet from sites such as the UCLA Pain Management Clinical Resource Guide, http://www.anes.ucla.edu/pain/assessment_tools.html. An example of an assessment tool is given in Table 6.5.

The problem with any behavioural assessment tool for infants and neonates is that it may not be applicable. If the child is premature, very ill or receiving sedating drugs, he or she may not demonstrate any behavioural response to pain at all. Pain assessment will then rely on the subjective judgement of the nurse or carer. Importantly though, the process of undertaking a pain assessment conveys important messages to the parents. It makes a statement that pain matters and is important in the overall care of the infant.

An example of a tool devised for children in the immediate postoperative period is the Children's Hospital of Eastern Ontario Pain Scale (CHEOPS) (McGrath et al. 1985). This is based on the categories of pain-related behaviours listed in Table 6.6. Pain behaviours are scored, the score being said to indicate distress. McGrath (1989) suggests that it is only distress that can be measured, as the tool has not been shown to demonstrate pure pain.

Given the plethora of tools currently in existence, it is easy to appreciate the difficulty in creating an assessment tool that meets all needs. Some may be useful in particular circumstances and for differing reasons, so assessment tools usually have to be individualised to suit the clinical circumstances.

The assumption that pain exists in preverbal children can only be just that, an assumption. We all know that many other factors can cause distress behaviour in small children. However, when distress is displayed in the context of a potentially painful condition, whether it is associated with disease, a painful procedure or follows injury or surgery, pain must always be considered to be the principal cause of this distress. Involving parents who have a close and intimate knowledge of how their children respond can make the job much easier. When pain may be the source of distress and the response of the infant is observed, analgesic protocols may be developed that help to ensure the timely and adequate management of pain.

Table 6.4 Examples of pain assessment tools and age range of infants tested

Tool	Age range
Pain Rating Scale (PRS) (Joyce et al. 1994)	Infants 1–12 months of age
Riley Infant Pain Scale (RIPS) (Schade et al. 1996)	Postoperative infants and children
Maximally Discriminative Facial Movement Coding System (MAX) (Izard 1995)	Infants 0–2 years
Infant Body Coding System (IBCS) (Craig et al. 1993)	Preterm and full-term newborns
Neonatal Pain and Discomfort Scale (EDIN) (Debillon et al. 2001)	Preterm infants, average gestational age 31.5 weeks
Clinical Scoring System (CSS) or Postoperative Pain Score (POPS) (Schade et al. 1996)	Infants from 1–7 months requiring surgery
Modified Postoperative Comfort Score (PCS) revision of POPS (Guinsburg et al. 1998)	Mechanically ventilated preterm infants
Behavioural Pain Score (Pokela 1994)	Mechanically ventilated preterm infants
Modified Behavioural Pain Scale (MBPS) (Taddio et al. 1995)	Healthy infants 4–6 months
Baby Facial Action Coding System (Baby FACS) (Rosenstein and Oster 1988)	Healthy newborns
Children's and Infants' Postoperative Pain Scale (CHIPPS) (Buttner and Finke 2002)	Newborns, infants and young children
Acute Pain Rating Scale for Neonates (Carbajal et al. 1997)	Newborns with gestational age 25–41 weeks
Liverpool Infant Distress Scale (LIDS) (Horgan and Choonara 1996)	Newborn infants postoperatively
Neonatal Facial Coding System (NFCS) (Grunau et al. 1998; Peters et al. 2003)	Preterm infants and well newborns
Bernese Pain Scale for Neonates (BPSN) (Cignacco et al. 2004)	Term and preterm neonates with and without CPAP ventilation
The Pain Assessment Tool (PATS) (Hodgkinson et al. 1994; Spence et al. 2005)	Neonates and critically ill ventilated infants in a neonatal intensive care unit
The Neonatal Pain Assessment Tool (Friedrichs et al. 1995)	Infants in an intensive care setting
The Scale for Use in Newborns (SUN) (Blauer and Gertsmann 1998)	Preterm and term infants during procedures
The Distress Scale for Ventilated Newborn Infants (DSVNI) (Sparshott 1996)	Initial reporting of tool development for newborns
The Comfort Scale (Ambuel et al. 1992; van Dijk et al. 2005)	Newborns to young children
The CRIES (Krechel and Bilner 1995)	Infants postoperatively
The Neonatal Infant Pain Scale (NIPS) (Lawrence et al. 1993; Hudson-Barr et al. 2002; Gallo 2003)	Preterm and term infants
The Pain Assessment in Neonates (PAIN) Scale (Hudson-Barr et al. 2002)	Neonates with gestational age 26–47 weeks
The Modified Infant Pain Scale (MIPS) (Buchholz et al. 1998)	Healthy term infants undergoing elective surgery
The Premature Infant Pain Profile (PIPP) (Stevens et al. 1996)	Newborns with gestational age 28–40 weeks
The Children's Hospital of Eastern Ontario Pain Scale (CHEOPS) (McGrath et al. 1985)	Neonates

Table 6.5 CRIES pain assessment tool

Parameter	Score		
	0	1	2
Crying	None	High pitched	Inconsolable
Requires O_2 to keep oxygen saturation > 95 per cent	No	<30%	>30%
Increased vital signs	HR and BP equal to or below preoperative values	HR and BP increased by <20 per cent over preoperative values	HR and BP increased by >20 per cent over preoperative values
Expression	None	Grimace	Grimace/grunt
Sleepless	No	Wakes at frequent intervals	Constantly awake

Source: Krechel and Bilner 1995

Table 6.6 CHEOPS assessment categories

- Crying
- Facial expression
- Verbalisation (both pain and non-pain related)
- Movement of the torso
- Tactile activity
- Leg movements

(McGrath et al. 1985)

Case history

Three-year-old James returned from theatre at 2 p.m. following a right orchipexy (open surgery for an undescended testicle). He was rousable but sleepy and both parents came with him back to the ward. His pain was being controlled via an intra-venous cannula, which could be used by the nurses following a protocol to adminis-ter intravenous opioid and non-opioid analgesia until oral medication could be tolerated. Observations were commenced and he seemed comfortable until about 3 p.m. when his heart rate increased and he became restless. The staff nurse looking after him decided to give him a dose of paracetamol and a couple of bolus doses of morphine according to the preprinted and signed analgesia prescription for acute pain in children (see Figure 6.1 for an example used in a district general hospital). His favourite cuddly toy was tucked under his arm and the radio played some soft music in the background. The lighting was dimmed enough to give the room a calm feel but sufficient for observations to take place. Ten minutes later James was sleeping comfortably and his observations were all within normal limits. When he woke up again half an hour later, he was able to sit up and have his tea, totally unconcerned by his operation.

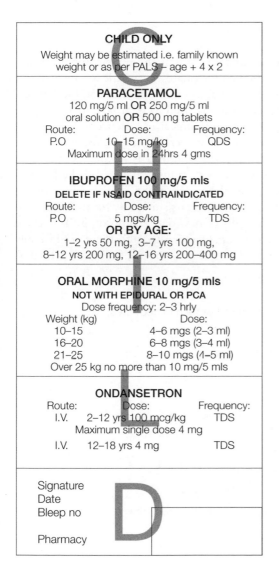

CHILD ONLY
Weight may be estimated i.e. family known
weight or as per PALS – age + 4 x 2

PARACETAMOL
120 mg/5 ml **OR** 250 mg/5 ml
oral solution **OR** 500 mg tablets
Route:	Dose:	Frequency:
P.O	10–15 mg/kg	QDS

Maximum dose in 24hrs 4 gms

IBUPROFEN 100 mg/5 mls
DELETE IF NSAID CONTRAINDICATED
Route:	Dose:	Frequency:
P.O	5 mgs/kg	TDS

OR BY AGE:
1–2 yrs 50 mg, 3–7 yrs 100 mg,
8–12 yrs 200 mg, 12–16 yrs 200–400 mg

ORAL MORPHINE 10 mg/5 mls
NOT WITH EPIDURAL OR PCA
Dose frequency: 2–3 hrly
Weight (kg)	Dose:
10–15	4–6 mgs (2–3 ml)
16–20	6–8 mgs (3–4 ml)
21–25	8–10 mgs (4–5 ml)

Over 25 kg no more than 10 mg/5 mls

ONDANSETRON
Route:	Dose:	Frequency:
I.V.	2–12 yrs 100 mcg/kg	TDS

Maximum single dose 4 mg
| I.V. | 12–18 yrs 4 mg | TDS |

Signature
Date
Bleep no

Pharmacy

Figure 6.1 Example of preprinted
analgesia prescription for acute pain
in children

Source: By kind permission of Poole Hospital
NHS Trust

Time out

The previous case history illustrates how a simple analgesia protocol can rapidly
reduce pain and stress. Can you think of some other pharmacological and non-
pharmacological strategies that may be useful to reduce pain and stress in the
very young child?

Pharmacological strategies

Pharmacological strategies may be similar to adults but as there are complex ethical problems with the study of drugs in children and neonates, very little is known about exactly which drugs are the most appropriate. Paracetamol, opioids and local anaesthetics are widely used. NSAIDs are less commonly used to treat postoperative pain in neonates, most likely due to lack of data and clinical experience. Topical local anesthetics such as EMLA (lidocaine and prilocaine) cream can be used for minor procedures, except heel lance and venipunctures. Caution is needed when using EMLA in young infants due to the toxic effects of transdermally absorbed anaesthetic. There are now also some concerns about morphine in the frail preterm neonate. For so long the traditional opioid of choice, its suitability for the ventilated neonate is beginning to be questioned in light of new data (Sampson 2007). Table 6.7 provides some guidelines on the use of analgesia. Although these could really apply to pain in any age group, they have been drawn up specifically for neonates, infants and children.

Table 6.7 General guidelines for the management of pain in neonates, infants and children

• Anticipate predictable painful experiences and intervene
• Involve the family
• Use multimodal approaches and treat early
• Analgesics should be administered on a schedule around the clock for moderate-to-severe pain rather than as needed
• Use intravenous medications for severe acute pain
• Oral medications are preferred for mild-to-moderate pain
• Base the initial choice of analgesia on the severity and type of pain
• Adjust the analgesic dose and dosing interval based on regular and systematic pain assessment
• Titrate the analgesic dose as necessary until pain relief is achieved, side effects become unmanageable or maximum recommended dosages are reached. There is no maximum dose for opioids unless given in combination with a drug such as paracetamol
• Monitor and manage any side effects. Side effects that can be anticipated such as constipation should be prevented or treated promptly
• When selecting an opioid, consider whether the patient is opioid naive or tolerant. Patients on opioids regularly for approximately seven days may require higher doses for acute pain control
• Provide rescue analgesia for breakthrough pain. Increase maintenance dose of opioid if more than two rescue doses per day are needed

Source: Adapted from the American Academy of Paediatrics and American Pain Society (2001) and Anand and the International Evidence-based Group for Neonatal Pain (2001)

Non-pharmacological strategies

Many of the traditional non-pharmacological strategies, especially psychological techniques, are applicable only to the fully verbal patient. Strategies such as information-giving or using positive imagery can hardly be applied to the newborn, but there are other therapies that might be of particular value, especially when used in combination with analgesia. These include:

- *Relieving the problem:* Could the pain possibly be alleviated by overcoming the cause? This may well be the most obvious and best solution, for example by splinting a painful limb, or inserting a nasogastric tube if abdominal distension might be causing discomfort.
- *Distraction therapy:* If possible, feeding during any procedure that may cause pain can be useful. This seems to be the case particularly with breastfeeding. Maternal smell may promote infant bonding and feelings of security and skin-to-skin contact has also been suggested as an important factor. Non-nutritive sucking on a dummy, or a dummy or cotton wool stick sprinkled with sucrose or distilled water has been shown to significantly reduce crying and pain responses in neonates undergoing heel lance procedures and circumcision (Stevens et al. 2004; South et al. 2005). It has been suggested that sucrose can stimulate the release of endogenous endorphins as, interestingly, analgesia appears to be reversed with the administration of naloxone (Kracke et al. 2005).
- *Relaxation therapy:* Gentle touch and massage may well be as beneficial to small children as it is to adults (Diego et al. 2005). Not only can massage relax and soothe, but as a form of cutaneous stimulation, it may also help to close the 'pain gate' referred to in Chapter 1.
- *Comfort strategies:* Keep the neonate warm and eliminate loud noise and bright light. Ensure that examination, nappy changes and turning are done at the same time, rather than constantly disturbing the neonate and causing further pain. Swaddling, facilitated tucking (where the infant's head and feet are cradled, with legs flexed and held close the trunk) and kangaroo care (involving infants held skin to skin with a parent) have also been shown to be of benefit (Golianu et al. 2007).
- *Cold therapy:* A refrigerant spray, for example, can cool an area prior to inserting a needle.
- *Acupuncture and acupressure:* These may also have some utility, particularly in the perioperative period or in a neonatal intensive care unit, although further studies are needed (Golianu et al. 2007).

For a systematic review on the efficacy of non-pharmacological interventions in the management of procedural pain in preterm and term infants, see Cignacco et al. (2007).

Much more research is needed, but at least we now have a better understanding of the neurological development of small children. The basic pharmacological principles are coming under more intense scrutiny. We also have some assessment tools to work with that are based on the observation of facial expressions and on behavioural and psychological measures. The education of healthcare professionals to dispel some long-held myths is still a priority, but at last the issue of pain in children and neonates is becoming a feature of contemporary research. The development of specialised pain assessment tools has been very helpful; it is now essential that they are utilised effectively in practice. Striving to improve our knowledge and involving parents and close relatives can be a positive step towards recognising and treating the pain experienced by some of the most vulnerable patients in our care.

Further reading

Duhn L. (2004) A systematic integrative review of infant pain assessment tools. *Advanced Neonatal Care*, 4(3): 126–40, Medscape, http://www.medscape.com/viewarticle/484129_10.

McKenzie I., Gaukroger P., Ragg P. and Brown T. (1997) *Manual of Acute Pain Management in Children*. London, Churchill Livingstone.

National Guideline Clearinghouse, *Prevention and Management of Pain in the Neonate: An Update*, http/:www.guideline.gov.

Ranger R., Johnston C. and Anand K. (2007) Current controversies regarding pain assessment in neonates. *Seminars in Perinatology,* 31: 283–8.

Sharek P., Powers R., Koehn A. and Anand J. (2006) Evaluation and development of potentially better practices to improve pain. *Pediatrics,* 118: S78–S86.

Thomas N. (ed.) (1997) *Pain: Its Nature and Management*. London, Baillière Tindall. (Specific chapters deal with the management of children's pain and management strategies for pain in the elderly.)

Ethnic minorities

The term 'ethnic minority' refers to a group of people who may not share the same language, culture, nationality, spiritual or religious beliefs as the majority. Since the late 1940s, researchers have been intrigued by the influence that cultural background may have on the experience and expression of pain. We are all aware that people respond quite differently to painful stimuli. Some may become extremely vocal and distressed following what appear to be relatively minor stimuli; while other individuals appear unconcerned by what seem to be extremely painful stimuli. A society may value and encourage stoicism, the British 'stiff upper lip' being a good example of how expectations may influence an individual's response. On the other hand, another culture may expect pain to be accompanied by a vigorous verbal and behavioural response. Subtle genetic differences are also suggesting that individual cultures may even differ biologically, with thresholds to pain varying as well as physiological responses to pain medication (Davidhizar and Giger 2004). Not only are there differences in how different cultural groups express their pain, there is evidence that the prevalence of pain may be different in diverse groups. For example, in a study undertaken in Greater Manchester (Allison et al. 2002), the prevalence of musculoskeletal pain was higher in people from ethnic minority groups than it was among white people. A selective literature review by experts revealed a disparity in the way people from different ethnic backgrounds are treated for their pain (Green et al. 2003).

Melzack and Wall's gate control theory and more recently Melzack's neuromatrix theory of pain (Chapter 1) have helped to provide an explanation for this variation in pain tolerance and expression. Cultural difference may substantially influence our response to pain as a result of us modelling our behaviour on how others, similar to us, have behaved. When we experience pain, we draw on this model, our pain behaviour somehow reflecting our cultural background. The research certainly seems to give these theories credence, with fascinating studies of very different reactions to painful encounters that to our Western eyes would seem too terrible to bear. A child in a large family who is brought up not to fear pain but to accept it as an inevitable part of life may react quite differently from an only child who has been cosseted and experienced a dramatic parental reaction to every small bruise and scratch.

In their book *The Challenge of Pain* (1996), Melzack and Wall discuss several cultures and the different ways in which certain people accept pain, often as part of a religious ceremony. Zborowski (1952) was the author of some key work that looked at the response to pain by groups of Irish, Italian and Anglo-American individuals, concluding that definite cultural differences could be predicted. Numerous other studies have been conducted, but the methodology and analysis of findings can be problematic when dealing with an experience as subjective as pain. However, research is also shedding some light on the significant differences that may be seen in drug metabolism, dosing requirements, therapeutic response and side effects in racial and ethnic groups (Salerno 1995).

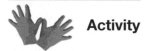 **Activity**

Have you nursed many patients from a cultural background different from your own who were expressing pain in a way you did not expect? If you have, make a few notes on how they were responding. Discuss these with an experienced colleague. Have they noted any differences in the way in which certain ethnic minorities respond to pain? Did these differences make pain assessment more challenging?

It would seem not only that culture and ethnic background influence an individual's response to pain, but there is also evidence that our own background can influence how we as nurses respond to others in pain. Davidhizar and Giger (2004) reported that nurses were influenced not just by cultural differences in patients, but also by their own cultural background, age and social class. Negative stereotyping can sometimes occur when we experience cultural practices or behaviour that differ from those regarded as our own cultural norm and this can reveal itself in ways such as opioid prescribing. A study in the USA indicated that white patients remain significantly more likely to receive an opioid for pain than black, Hispanic or Asian patients (Sherwood et al. 2005).

Childbirth and pain have been studied extensively. Some carers may feel that pain is a part of childbirth and does not require much intervention but this view may be totally in conflict with that of the woman in labour. Unfortunately, negative stereotyping is also encountered when carers and patients hold conflicting views. A small-scale ethnographic study undertaken by Bowler (1993) looked at the experience of childbirth in mothers of South Asian descent and discussed the stereotypical views held by some midwives, which revealed four main themes:

- difficulty in communication
- the women's lack of compliance with the care available and their abuse of the service
- their tendency to 'make a fuss about nothing'
- their lack of 'normal maternal instinct'.

Women with little English were branded as 'rude and unintelligent', some midwives expressing the view that language difficulties were 'the patients' problem'. From this study, it can clearly be seen that difficulties with healthcare for ethnic minorities can be experienced because of a lack of understanding of or sensitivity to the effects that background can have on how we deal with pain and stress. Like so many of the challenges that pain may bring to care, when communication is a problem, there is evidence that nurses may experience negative feelings, may distance themselves from the patient or may limit themselves to giving 'physical' or 'routine' care (Forrest 1989).

If a culture values stoicism in the face of pain and hardship, adjusting to individuals inclined to respond to pain publicly or vocally can lead to conflict and negative stereotyping, an issue that clearly needs to be addressed. A fascinating study by Harper et al. (2007) explored how military trained nurses rationalised their postoperative pain management decisions and how these differed from the patients' self-reports. The study highlights how the socialisation of nurses in a military culture can influence the complexity of pain management.

Our cultural background may influence every aspect of our experience of pain from how we react, what treatment we seek and the intensity and duration of the pain we tolerate, to when we report pain, whom we report it to and what type of pain requires attention (Meinhart and McCaffery 1983). Understanding this cultural influence on pain will prepare us better to cope with a response that is either unexpected or alarming when placed in the context of our own beliefs and culture.

Incorporating the following simple strategies can assist in responding to pain across cultures (Davidhizar and Giger 2004):

- Utilise an appropriate assessment tool that if necessary has been translated or adapted for a particular cultural group
- Appreciate variations in response to pain
- Be sensitive to variations in communication styles
- Recognise that communicating pain may not be acceptable behaviour within a particular culture

- Utilise knowledge of biological variations to painful stimuli and responses to medication
- Develop a personal awareness of values and beliefs, which may affect responses to pain.

Further reading

Green C., Anderson K., Baker T., Campbell L., Becker S. et al. (2003) The unequal burden of pain: confronting racial and ethnic disparities in pain. *Pain Medicine*, 4: 277–9.
Morris D. (1993) *The Culture of Pain*. Berkeley, CA, University of California Press.
Parsons, E.P. (1992) Cultural aspects of pain. *Surgical Nurse*, 5(2): 14–16.

Conclusion

The observation of visual or behavioural indicators of pain is only useful when incorporated into a systematic strategy of observation, planning and regular evaluation. Although we lack the perfect assessment tools for particularly vulnerable patients, we also lack a culture of regular pain assessment. Regular assessment is vital if we are going to be able effectively to trial a therapy and evaluate its effect. Evaluation is the final and most critical step in managing pain. The evaluation of any strategies can only be based on careful monitoring, and for that one needs a basic observation strategy that enables observed signs of possible pain to be documented and treatments evaluated in light of these documented observations.

For cognitively impaired or immature groups of patients, analgesia may be especially hard to evaluate, and many of the psychological strategies to improve pain relief require a high level of cognitive function, something that will be lacking in this group of patients. The situation is, however, improving and the further reading at the end of each section will direct you to more in-depth texts.

Where language and culture create barriers to effective pain management, more thought may perhaps be given to extending the role of interpreters and encouraging a greater involvement of the family. The inclusion of cultural studies in both pre- and postregistration education will help to raise the awareness of possible problems and conflicts. Preparing healthcare professionals to deal effectively with potential misunderstandings may ultimately reduce their impact on patient care.

After a break, try the multiple choice test below in order to self-assess your learning so far. For some of the questions, more than one answer will be correct, however, there will be one answer that is so far best supported by the evidence.

Managing Pain in Vulnerable Patients
Multiple choice TEST

1. Historically, pain management in neonates has been neglected. What is the main reason for this?
    a. A lack of reliable and valid pain assessment tools
    b. A belief that neonates do not feel pain
    c. A significant lack of research available to guide practice development
    d. The fact that treatment for pain using opioids was risky and therefore best avoided

2. At what stage of development are the endorphin and inhibitory systems thought to be fully functional in the neonate?
    a. 3rd trimester
    b. At 12 weeks old
    c. At term
    d. At birth

3. Which of the following drugs, although used extensively, has recently been causing a little more concern when used for the very frail premature neonate?
    a. Paracetamol
    b. Alfentanyl
    c. Morphine
    d. Fentanyl

4. Which pain assessment tool do you feel could be the most effective for use with the cognitively impaired elderly?
    a. A visual analogue scale
    b. A verbal rating
    c. A behavioural rating score
    d. A pain diary

5. When developing an assessment tool based on behaviour, how can individual assessor bias be avoided?
    a. By only having one assessor
    b. By always incorporating an objective measurement, for example pulse or blood pressure
    c. By making sure that everyone is well trained and attends an education session
    d. By ensuring that the tool possesses explicit criteria for measurement

6. For patients with learning disability or a brain injury, which of the following strategies for assessing pain is likely to be the most helpful?
    a. Observing patients for distress
    b. Having a detailed personal profile available
    c. Monitoring physiological indicators of distress
    d. Asking the nurse caring for the patient most often if they think the patient is in pain

7. Whom do you feel would be the most accurate in assessing pain in cognitively impaired patients who cannot communicate verbally?
    a. Doctors
    b. Nurses
    c. Healthcare assistants
    d. Relatives

8. Correctly matching the source of pain with its type, which of the following is the more common?
   a. Shingles infection *and* postherpetic neuralgia ☐
   b. Diabetes *and* visceral pain ☐
   c. Musculoskeletal injury *and* ischaemic pain ☐
   d. Cancer *and* small joint pain ☐

9. Which of the following is a poor indicator of chronic pain in an adult patient unable to communicate?
   a. An alteration in blood pressure ☐
   b. Facial expression ☐
   c. Altered social interaction ☐
   d. A change in posture ☐

10. When cognitively impaired patients experience an acute injury, when should they receive analgesia?
   a. When they show obvious signs of distress ☐
   b. Whenever they display changes in behaviour or facial expression ☐
   c. On a regular basis, based on the duration of action of the drug ☐
   d. When they are moved or have a procedure done to them ☐

Answers

1. c. A significant lack of research available to guide practice development; until research began to be published, there was little evidence to convince clinicians that practice needed to change. This evidence did not start to emerge until the mid-1980s. Although the development of reliable and valid pain assessment tools was imperative for the effective management of pain, this was not the main factor involved. For many years, it was a widely held belief that neonates did not have the neural development to feel pain, so pain management was not deemed necessary; this has only fairly recently been disproved. Treatment for pain in neonates using opioids was risky and therefore best avoided, although this was a factor that discouraged clinicians from prescribing and administering opioids; again, however, it was not the main reason.

2. a. 3rd trimester.

3. c. Morphine; although all drugs must be given cautiously in the very frail preterm neonate. There are major concerns that most pain medications, particularly opioids, have not been tested in neonates and therefore there is a lack of research to assist clinicians. Opioids routinely form part of analgesia regimes for neonates but new research is vital to ensure the safest drug regimes are used and readers need to keep up to date with the latest findings.

4. b. A verbal rating; despite their cognitive impairment, many patients can still tell you they are in pain and how bad it is. Few would be able to manage a visual analogue scale. Behaviour rating scores can be useful for the totally non-communicative and a pain diary, although beyond the ability of the patient to maintain, may have some utility if this was completed by staff or carers. However, the reality is this is unlikely to happen.

5. d. By ensuring that it possesses explicit criteria for measurement; clear criteria will reduce the chance of assessor bias and improve the reliability of the scale. Only having one assessor might reduce the chance of error between assessors, but it is not practical and the assessor would still need to know what to look for to rate the pain. Although it might be useful to incorporate an objective measurement, for example pulse or blood pressure, it is important that scales do not rely solely on one dimension of expression; again, this would not be practical. Making sure that everyone is well trained and attends an education session is important and would help, but it is not the prime answer as people could still make their own interpretations.

6. b. Having a detailed personal profile available. Although observing for distress or the physiological indicators of distress are important, unless you know how the patient is likely to specifically manifest pain distress from a profile, you may run into problems and miss unique pain indicators. Unfortunately, healthcare professionals have not consistently been shown to be able to identify pain in those unable to communicate. Certainly, the nurse who spends the most time with a patient, especially if they are experienced in observing pain behaviour, will be helpful.

7. d. Relatives would appear to be better than all healthcare professionals at assessing pain in patients who cannot communicate. Parents with severely brain-injured children seem especially able to pick up signals of pain and discomfort that to an outsider are extremely subtle and difficult to identify.

8. a. Shingles infection and postherpetic neuralgia is correct. Viruses of the herpes family can lie dormant in nerves, shingles being an example that can lead to postherpetic neuralgia. Diabetes most commonly results in neuropathic pain, usually beginning in the hands and feet, although in more advanced cases, visceral pain can develop. Musculoskeletal problems such as osteoporosis cause fractures and contractures but are unlikely to be implicated in vascular ischaemic pain. Cancer pain elicits a range of pain types but not specifically small joint pain; the latter would be more typical of arthritis.

9. a. An alteration in blood pressure is physiologically demanding, and once pain is no longer acute, the body adapts. Chronic pain can often elicit no obvious pathological changes. Observations of facial expression, altered social interaction and change in posture have all been used to assess pain.

10. c. On a regular basis, based on the duration of action of the drug, would seem to be the most humane method, combined with regular assessment and evaluation to ensure that the medication is working, is still needed and is not producing side effects. This will obviously require a great deal of skill, but given that all the evidence, especially surrounding the elderly and cognitively impaired, indicates that we have managed pain very badly in the past, pre-empting any obvious signs of pain for a few days seems sensible. Unfortunately, the effective observation of behavioural signs for assessment purposes is only just being developed.

CHAPTER 7

Nursing Patients with Challenging Pain

Learning outcomes

On completion of this chapter, the student will be able to:

- Identify two groups of clients for whom pain management will be particularly challenging
- Discuss factors that contribute to pain being inadequately or inappropriately managed for these people
- Critically analyse the challenging aspects related to pain management for an individual you have cared for
- Evaluate strategies that might lead to improved pain relief for the individual selected above

Indicative reading

British Pain Society (2007) *Pain and Substance Misuse: Improving the Patient Experience*. London, British Pain Society, http://www.britishpainsociety.org/book_drug_misuse_main.pdf.

De Jong A., Middlekoop E., Faber A. and Van Loey N. (2007) Non-pharmacological nursing interventions for procedural pain relief in adults with burns: a systematic literature review. *Burns*, 33(7): 811–27.

Finnerup N. and Jensen T. (2004) Spinal cord injury pain: mechanisms and treatment. *European Journal of Neurology*, 11: 73–82.

Marlowe K. (2002) Treatment of sickle cell pain. *Pharmacotherapy*, 22(4): 484–91, Medscape, http://www.medscape.com/viewarticle/432395_1.

Oyama O., Paltoo C. and Greengold J. (2007) Somatoform disorders. *American Family Physician*, 76(9): 1333–8.

Background

Although pain is an individual and unique experience, previous chapters on the management of acute and chronic pain have considered the 'normal' pattern of events. This chapter captures a range of pain experiences that have received relatively scant attention in the literature but, as in the vulnerable patient, often present a considerable challenge to clinicians. While we may not offer the answers here, we hope to raise your awareness, stimulate a dialogue and provide reference material, relevant articles and supportive ideas.

The need for a chapter such as this stems from a growing demand from the public for healthcare to define a cause for a disorder, especially a painful one, treat the cause and solve the problem. Unfortunately, for many in society, the symptom of pain is not so straightforward, but success in other spheres of healthcare fuels the demand to cure all ills. We now live in a society that has high expectations of what healthcare can deliver, and those in pain are no longer prepared to suffer in silence. However, when we are faced with pain that challenges our ability to relieve it or, even in some cases, understand it, the encounter can be frustrating and unsatisfactory for staff and patients alike. The term 'heart-sink' sometimes springs to mind when one is left to confront the patient with mountainous notes for whom no interventions or therapy have so far appeared to offer any control of pain or relief of suffering.

We first consider the care of patients with particularly challenging pain, those whose pain follows serious burns and those with spinal injuries. Then we look at people with sickle-cell disease, who can experience intense, life-threatening pain crises, which are often inadequately relieved. Mood disorders, examined next, can be powerful in altering our perception of pain and coping strategies. Substance misuse is a huge social issue, and the management of pain in patients with a history of substance misuse can pose particular challenges when they enter the healthcare system. Lastly, we cover those patients whose pain may be associated with secondary gain, which, although not consciously sought, can be significant in terms of the part it can play in their recovery. Each section of the chapter outlines the issues and makes suggestions on strategies to improve pain management. It is assumed that the assessment of pain is a necessary prerequisite prior to the selection of any interventions, and you may at some time wish to refer back to Chapter 2.

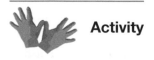 **Activity**

Go to the library and look up substance misuse, burns and spinal injuries in the index of several contemporary pain textbooks. How many books actually contained text related to these problems?

It is likely that very few of these issues appeared in a textbook or, if they did, they were mentioned in passing. Another way of considering the scope of a topic is to look at the contents page of a book and work out how many pages are actually dedicated to the topic you are interested in and what percentage of the book they form.

It is helpful to consider how the topics we are going to explore fit within the multidimensional framework of pain. Two main categories of pain can be defined by their cause: is the pain based on a pathophysiological disorder or a psychological disorder driven by disordered perception and behaviour? Figure 7.1, although simplistic, offers an illustration of the physical and psychological influences on pain; as in reality, pain is a complex mixture of both categories. It may be helpful therefore to view pain as a continuum, with physical causes at one end and psychosocial influences at the other. Although **psychogenic** pain is quite rare (Covington 2000), the role of psychological factors in chronic or disabling pain are well recognised. What we now know about the development of chronic pain is that approximately one-half to two-thirds of all patients diagnosed with chronic pain manifest various levels of psychosocial distress (Manchikanti et al. 2002). A significant proportion will be diagnosed with reactive disorders including depression, anxiety, somatisation disorder, and personality disorders experienced with a background of emotional issues such as anger, frustration and loss of self-esteem (Gatchel and Epkar 1999). When we add in the powerful influences of the stress response, perhaps a violent or abusive past and genetic vulnerability to pain, we can see how challenging pain relief can prove to be for certain groups of patients. It might also be useful here to refer back to Chapter 1 for an overview of the theories of pain.

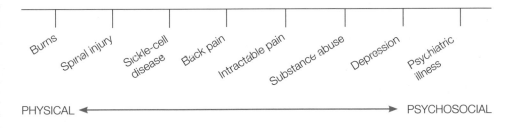

Figure 7.1 Physical and psychological influences on pain

Pain following a serious burn

People who have experienced burns have several needs, all of which impact on their experience of pain. Pain management is an essential and an integral part of their nursing care yet pain has a poor record of being managed effectively (Summer et al. 2007). This section will consider why people who have been burnt have special needs, as well as other key aspects of their pain management.

The pain of a burn is known to us all. We have all at one time or another been unfortunate enough to catch our hand on a cooker, in a fire, in steam or with boiling water. It used to be assumed that the larger the area of burn, the greater the pain, and the deeper the burn, the less pain because of the nerve endings being destroyed within the deeper damaged tissues. In practice, most deep burn areas are intermingled with damage to superficial tissue, and pain is usually a definite sequela. A burn may also damage tissue irreparably, resulting in long-term disfigurement and anguish from these scars. The emotional turmoil can contribute significantly to the experience of pain.

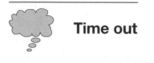 **Time out**

Have you ever had a serious burn, or do you know someone who has experienced one? What was the pain like? Did the pain change over time? Was pain related to any particular activity?

It was likely that the pain was initially intense and sharp but that the administration of cold (usually running) water then reduced the pain sensation. Later, a deep throbbing pain might have emerged, along with anxiety about the consequences of the burn and how it would heal. Day-to-day background discomfort is there most of the time, and it may be painful to move the affected limb. It should be remembered that many burns involve children, and it has already been described how their pain is often neglected and presents the practitioner with additional challenges related to assessment (see Chapter 6).

Changing the dressing

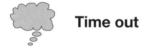 **Time out**

When you take a sticking plaster off, how do you feel? Imagine that the sticking plaster has stuck to your burn or cut, and a friend comes along and offers to help to rip the tape off. What do you say?

It is likely that the initial pain you experience when you come to take the plaster off makes you anxious about the pain you predict you will feel. If a friend offers to remove it for you, you will probably decline (most kindly, of course), as you will prefer to have control of this pain-eliciting activity yourself.

In clinical situations, we often take this control away from patients by not allowing them to participate in their dressing changes. Research with burns patients has demonstrated that by allowing them to exert some control over their own dressing changes, they experience significantly less pain (Sutherland 1996). It has also been shown that reducing the number of times the dressing is changed can reduce the pain associated with dressing change. Sheridan et al. (1997) undertook a research study with 50 burned children and found that a once-daily change resulted in no significant alteration in infection morbidity compared with twice-daily changing.

Madjar (1998) has written an excellent book on her own research, which explores the lived experience of pain inflicted in the context of medically prescribed treatment. Based on interviews with burns patients and those receiving chemotherapy, she explores the infliction of pain from the perspective of patients and nurses. Without an understanding of inflicted pain, nurses are ill prepared to reduce the incidence or prevalence of such pain or manage their own feelings of stress when they have to inflict pain. It is a thought-provoking book that helps us to understand rather than feel guilty.

Psychosocial interventions

The devastating nature of a burn increases the psychological and physiological responses of the person involved. Traumatic stress disorders associated with burn injury have been reported to be as high as 50% (Esselman et al. 2006). Although the pain of burns can be treated reasonably effectively by aggressive and multimodal analgesic interventions, it is the inclusion of psychological strategies that can enhance the effectiveness of pain management and improve recovery.

Case history

Peter is an 18-year-old student who sustained a major burn to his back following an incident with a bonfire and fireworks when his clothes caught fire. He is currently on a surgical ward and is facing his first dressing change without a general anaesthetic. It is critical to manage pain and anxiety aggressively for the first dressing change to lessen the fear of subsequent procedures; therefore the following multimodal approach is taken. Peter is already using a PCA with 1mg morphine and a five-minute lockout, which has been working quite well. He is encouraged to use this as needed and is given reassurance that the nurse looking after him can administer additional bolus doses should these be necessary. This is done using a pre-agreed protocol by a nurse trained in the titration of intravenous opioids. Peter has also been receiving regular oral paracetamol and gabapentin to reduce hyperalgesia and opioid consumption. Prior to the dressing change, this is supplemented with low dose intravenous ketarolac. Peter is also offered the use of Entonox, which he declines, having found that it made him nauseous when he used it in the ambulance.

Prior to this dressing change, Peter has been given instructions on using relaxation and imagery techniques to help control procedural pain and he has been practising these with the acute pain nurse during one of her visits. He also accepts the offer of headphones so he can listen to relaxing music during the dressing change. He finds the staff are gentle, trustworthy and sensitive, they display technical competence and communicate with confidence and skill, which he finds reassuring. They tell Peter that if he asks them to stop the procedure they will do so for a short break, which gives him a sense of control. Although very busy, they adopt an 'unhurried' approach and the first dressing is changed with pain reduced to a minimum. Although unpleasant, Peter is left feeling that his pain can be controlled and he faces future dressing changes without excessive fear. After the PCA is discontinued, the opioid content of Peter's analgesia is replaced with oral transmucosal fentanyl in the form of a compressed lozenge on a stick that can be absorbed rapidly through the buccal mucosa. Although developed and licensed for use by patients with terminal disease, this works well with the additional non-opioid and non-pharmacological strategies.

Pharmacological therapy is of course absolutely vital for both background and procedural pain and usually comprises a combination of opioids, sometimes combined with anxiolytics (drugs used to treat anxiety) for painful procedures, NSAIDs, local anaesthetics and/or adjuvants such as the anticonvulsant gabapentin (Cuignet et al. 2007) or ketamine (Murat 2003).

Although protocols and guidelines have been developed, the intensity of pain associated with wound care and rehabilitation will vary widely over the long course of burn recovery, making effective pain management extremely challenging.

Psychological strategies

Useful psychological strategies include cognitive and behavioural interventions. If the patient is unable to move easily, the use of a video or music for distraction can be helpful. Recent research using computer-generated 'virtual reality' (VR) has shown some promising outcomes for patients having their burn dressings changed (van Twillert et al. 2007). Pain and anxiety were reduced through the use of VR and TV during dressing changes.

Think about where the dressing changes take place. If the unit has a specific 'room', what could be done to make this a pleasant environment that might take someone's mind off the pain? If the walls are plain, how about inviting an artist in to create some murals? This could be done in partnership with the patients as they might have some ideas too. Can you play music, computer games, use VR or have the TV available? Don't forget the ceiling – a mobile or pictures can be more interesting than a blank space.

Nowadays, there are also catalogues available that contain many items of distraction therapy from equipment, toys and special interactive books, to bubble tubes and so on, from which everyone can benefit. Most of these are targeted at children and those with learning difficulties, either to stimulate their environment or to distract attention away from something that is potentially unpleasant. Snoezelen – a sensory environment purported to produce relaxation and usually used for chronic pain – may also be a way of providing distraction (Schofield 2002).

From personal experience, when dealing with children, it can be useful to keep interactive, distracting toys and therapies in a special box, to be used only when an inflicted pain of short duration is unavoidable. The use of these distracting toys can have a 'knock-on' benefit that is not just confined to the child. The child playing with interactive toys can distract and calm an anxious parent who may be subconsciously transmitting his or her fear and apprehension to the child. For adults and children alike, it can be worthwhile using visually distracting strategies such as snoezelen, lava lamps and fibreoptic lamps that constantly change colour, as well as any equipment that will project all sorts of colours, lights and images onto the walls and ceilings. In this high-tech world, the use of virtual reality games may be of particular benefit especially for children and adolescents (Hoffman et al. 2001).

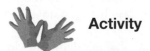 **Activity**

Next time you have to carry out an activity on a patient that might cause some discomfort, try using some form of distraction. For example, if the procedure is to be undertaken on a child, try getting somebody to read from a large book that obscures the child's view of what you are doing. If possible, get the child to suck on a boiled sweet at the same time. Remember that sucrose on a dummy sucked by a baby can reduce the crying time of babies having a needle stick (Lewindon et al. 1998). Conversation with adults can focus on recalling pleasant memories such as a recent holiday or a favourite place.

Further reading

Summer G., Puntillo K., Miaskowski C., Green P. and Levine J. (2007) Burn injury pain: the continuing challenge. *Journal of Pain*, 8(7): 533–48.

Pain in the patient with a spinal injury

The effective management of pain continues to be a significant problem in people with spinal cord injuries, but until recently there was little agreement on the definitions of the different types of pain following such trauma. The International Association for the Study of Pain has now set up a spinal cord injury pain task force proposing a new taxonomy, which is gaining acceptance (Siddall et al. 2000). This has been very helpful, particularly as recent studies indicate that approximately two-thirds of all spinal cord injury patients suffer from chronic pain and in one-third of these the pain is severe (Siddall et al. 2002). Not only does this interfere with rehabilitation and quality of life, the pain may be so severe that it leads to depression and even suicide in some of these patients (Widerstrom-Noga et al. 2001).

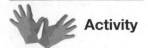 **Activity**

Why do you think this might be, and what implications could this have for people with spinal cord injuries?

Research summary

Finnerup and Jensen (2004) have written a review that provides some insight into the mechanisms of spinal cord injury pain. The article suggests some pharmacological treatments, which emphasise the importance of the distinction between nociceptive and neuropathic pain.

Nociceptive pain describes musculoskeletal pain including bone, joint and muscle trauma or inflammation, pain from mechanical instability, muscle spasm and secondary overuse syndromes particularly in the arms and shoulders of patients following a lower spinal cord injury. In addition, visceral pain may be a feature caused by kidney stones, bowel and sphincter dysfunction and headache.

Neuropathic pain can arise from three levels:

- above the level of the injury – compression neuropathy such as **carpel tunnel syndrome** and **complex regional pain syndrome**
- at the level of injury – nerve root compression, **syringomyelia**, spinal cord trauma and ischaemia, dual level cord and root trauma
- below the level of injury – spinal cord trauma and ischaemia (Siddall et al. 2000; Finnerup and Jensen 2004).

Although most patients will probably experience a mix of pain following spinal injury, the distinction is made between the two different pathophysiological causes of pain in the person with a spinal cord injury because the pharmacological targets are quite different. Pain resulting from tissue damage to skin, viscera, bone and so on usually responds well to analgesia, while neuropathic pain caused by damage to the nervous system may not. Neuropathic pain is complex because it results from pathological changes in the nervous system, which can be central or peripheral. Interventions aimed at interfering with traditional pain pathways, for example NSAIDS and opioids, may be ineffective. Neuropathic pain may be generated from damage to peripheral nerves or to the central nervous system, sometimes referred to as 'central pain'. Many patients with neuropathic pain complain of burning or icy pain, some have allodynia (pain elicited by light touch). The treatment of neuropathic pain has relied on drugs such as antidepressants (for example amitriptyline) and anticonvulsants that inhibit central mechanisms (for example gabapentin). While these are the preferred pharmacological strategies for most neuropathic pain, they have proved somewhat disappointing for spinal cord injury pain. Lignocaine showed promise when given intravenously but this was not sustained with the oral version mexiletine. Surprisingly, opioids may be useful in certain patients, as may ketamine (Backonja and Serra 2004). Because of the different mechanisms of pain involved in spinal cord injury, combining pharmacological with non-pharmacological therapy appears to offer the most effective treatment. So far, massage, which may have the added benefit of reducing depression and anxiety in this very at-risk group, and heat have been rated as effective for pain relief. TENS and acupuncture may provide some benefit for a subgroup of patients as well as physical exercise. Now we have a classification of pain based on underlying mechanisms, this will hopefully help to target treatment more effectively in the future.

Living with a spinal injury

 Time out

Why is it so important that pain in the person with a spinal injury is managed effectively?

Several reasons emerge, despite the challenges that pain management for these patients poses. Survivors are often grappling with multiple injuries and may have been fortunate to escape death. This life-changing circumstance is accompanied by a turmoil of emotions. The advent of pain in an area of their body that they can no longer feel, or use as they previously did, can cause anxiety and possibly hope (that this signals healing). It may also be difficult to understand as the physiology is complex, and if healthcare professionals dismiss their pain, sufferers may feel isolated, vulnerable and angry. The medical treatment of spinal cord injuries has considerably increased life expectancy, and the experience of living with chronic pain should not be the reward for survival.

Quality of life is a critical factor for the survivor of an injury. Wagner Anke et al. (1995) found, unsurprisingly, that reduced quality of life and psychological distress were more prevalent in patients with pain than in those without pain. Jonathan Cole (2004), a neurophysiologist, interviewed people with spinal cord injuries and wrote a book, *Still Lives*, which explored the many dimensions of life following such an event. The book captures people who changed their lives and made sense of their new sensations as well as people for whom life stopped and adjustment was difficult. For some people, pain and adjustment to pain are a constant part of life. These poignant narratives enrich our understanding of life for people after a spinal cord injury and bring new understanding. Pain will obviously impair an individual's ability to cope with the severe impairment of these devastating injuries, and its effective management should, from the beginning, be integral to the plan of care for these people.

Further reading

Backonja M. and Serra J. (2004) Pharmacologic management Part 2: Lesser studied neuropathic pain diseases. *Pain Medicine*, 5(S1): 48–59.
Norrbrink Budh C. and Lundeberg T. (2004) Non-pharmacological pain-relieving therapies in individuals with spinal cord injury: a patient perspective. *Complementary Therapies in Medicine*, 12: 189–97.

Pain in patients with sickle-cell disease

Sickle-cell disease is the result of a group of genetic blood disorders characterised by a gene mutation that leads to the production of an abnormal haemoglobin (HbS). The shape of this haemoglobin is different because of its 'sickle' shape, which can lead to clumping of the cells during a 'crisis', causing extreme pain as they block the fine capillaries. Sickle-cell disease occurs more commonly in people (or their descendants) from parts of Africa and the Caribbean but it also occurs in people of other ethnicities such as southern European. In the UK, the incidence of sickle-cell disease is increasing steadily (Streetley 1997). The advent of a painful crisis is the most common symptom and is responsible for the second greatest number of emergency admissions to hospital in London.

Despite the pain associated with this disease being difficult to treat, it is suggested that once hospitalised, pain management should be fast, aggressive and closely monitored (Johnson 2004). Most guidelines also stress the need for opioids when pain is very severe, when a patient is admitted to hospital and when non-opioid analgesia alone has failed to relieve the pain. Unfortunately, poor education leads to ineffective or inappropriate pain management and contemporary guidelines are not always followed. In a review of available textbooks, only 4 (21%) of 19 medical textbooks are consistent with guidelines. Moreover, only 7 texts (37%) note that addiction is infrequent in this population (Solomon 2008).

Sickle-cell disease affects individuals from the moment they are born and is life-long. Survival is more precarious in the first five years of life and again at around 20–24 years of age, and life expectancy is around 40 years. The highest mortality occurs in the under-six age group, usually as a result of infection, which precipitates a crisis. Despite this being a serious and painful disease, many patients have experienced inconsistent and often inadequate treatments (Todd et al. 2006).

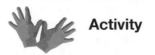 **Activity**

Find out which group of patients are usually affected by this disease. In your community, do you encounter sufferers of this disease and if so how are their health needs addressed?

This chronic disease can profoundly affect both sufferers and their families. They live with the uncertainty of the disease and the fear of a 'painful crisis', which can not only result in severe pain and illness, but also affect psychological well-being and ultimately prove fatal. Because of the prevalence of the disease within a culture that is often different from that of most healthcare professionals, these people sometimes feel neglected and disbelieved, their needs going unmet. In particular, the attitude of the healthcare professional can profoundly influence the effectiveness of pain management.

Living with sickle-cell disease

 Time out

Imagine what it might be like to have sickle-cell disease. How might your early experiences of a painful crisis affect you later in life?

Our experience of pain is affected by many variables, previous experience being just one of them. If you have been repeatedly admitted to hospital and your pain has not been managed effectively, you will probably feel very anxious when you have to return. This anxiety, pain and frustration will probably affect the way in which you behave towards the hospital staff. You may feel alienated and misunderstood or disbelieved. It may still be the case that in some areas, the pain of sickle-cell disease is exacerbated by prejudice as it usually affects black and poor people, whereas healthcare providers are usually white and middle class (see Chapter 6).

To ensure that a painful crisis is managed effectively, it is essential that healthcare professionals can assess pain accurately and establish a real belief in a patient's pain.

Case history

Henry is a 17-year-old Afro-Caribbean boy who arrives in A&E complaining of severe pain, which he says, is a result of a sickle-cell crisis. He tells the medical staff that when this has happened in the past, he has received 30mg morphine intravenously before the pain has begun to settle. They have no previous records and the patient is not carrying any sort of card or record from his previous hospital admissions. Morphine is ordered 10–15mg iv and the nurse starts to give it following the normal hospital protocol for intravenous opioid infusion. The patient asks that it be given rapidly and in one 'hit'. The nurse refuses to do this. Although Henry is a little more comfortable after the full 15mg have been administered, after an hour he requests another dose. He is still in severe pain and becomes angry and aggressive. The nurse does not believe that he is in the pain he states and feels that she is being used to obtain an opioid for its euphoric effects rather than pain relief. Conflict all round. The nurse feels frustrated because she has a moral and legal obligation to relieve pain and suffering but also a duty of care to avoid the administration of unnecessary medications.

This situation may perhaps be avoided with the advent of the electronic patient record, which should make access to previous care regimes more straightforward. The drugs and dosages that have been used effectively in the past can be recalled, along with a record of any previous or potential misuse risk. Maybe even a patient-held record could be used to help inform healthcare professionals of who the normal care provider is and what the 'usual' medication regime entails. Computerised records data from the European Haemoglobinopathy Registry – a collaborative multicentre registry for all patients with haemoglobinopathies – could be a big step forward (De 2005; European Haemoglobinopathy Registry 2006).

The experiences of Henry are far from unusual. Studies have generally found that healthcare professionals overestimate the prevalence of addiction in the sickle-cell disease population and these attitudes can have a negative and dehumanising effect, making the pain more severe and extending recovery times. Frequent doses of opioids to initially control pain during a crisis are not that unusual and close monitoring can help to detect adverse side effects in a group of patients who may have developed quite a high tolerance to opioids. As with most pain, do not overlook the role of a multimodal approach, combining analgesia to increase pain relief while reducing the side effects of large doses of any one medication.

The role of non-pharmacological therapies is, as always, important, such as cognitive behavioural therapy, distraction with TV and video games, biofeedback techniques, massage, relaxation, hypnotherapy and so on. To these strategies should be included advice on genetics, psychosocial counselling, preventive healthcare information and advice based on the identification of specific stressors that can trigger further attacks (De 2005).

Research summary

Much of the research so far conducted with patients suffering from sickle-cell disease exposes dissatisfaction with the management of their pain crises. Some of the difficulties, for example not being believed and having to wait for analgesia, are familiar problems for other groups of patients too. Sufferers report feeling isolated by their experience of 'crisis' pain, not being listened to, a lack of understanding from non-specialist clinicians, feeling they have a low priority, that their pain is invisible, they feel mistrusted by medical and nursing staff and social support networks are limited. All these negative feelings may lead to maladaptive coping, anger, aggression and the active avoidance of healthcare services (Booker et al. 2006).

In an attempt to address the difficulties faced by people in sickle-cell crisis, a dedicated day hospital in New York was created with the aim being to reduce pain and where possible prevent admission to hospital (Benjamin et al. 2000). Both these objectives were achieved and the hospital continues as a beacon of good practice. Finding new and creative ways to deliver services is essential to ensure that people with complex and challenging pain are managed appropriately.

It is important to have guidelines available to assist with treatment. The American Pain Society (1999) has developed a series of recommendations for the treatment of patients with sickle-cell disease and a synopsis of these is given in Table 7.1.

Table 7.1 A guide to the management of sickle-cell disease pain

- Pain management should be aggressive to ease pain and improve function
- Analgesics should be tailored to each patient. NSAIDs or paracetamol should be used to manage mild-to-moderate pain, unless contraindicated. If pain persists, an opioid should be added
- Because pethidine is toxic to the central nervous system, it should not be used if frequent large doses or long treatment durations are anticipated. (NB The use of this drug has now been severely curtailed in some countries)
- Opioid tolerance and physical dependence are expected with long-term opioid treatment and should not be confused with psychological dependence
- Sedatives and anxiolytics should not be used alone to manage pain because they can mask the behavioural response to pain without providing analgesia
- Severe pain should be considered a medical emergency, and timely and aggressive management should be provided until the pain becomes tolerable
- Equianalgesic (comparable analgesics given at doses required to achieve the equivalent pain relief) doses of oral opioids should be prescribed for home use when necessary
- Appropriate tapering of opioids in patients at risk for withdrawal syndromes is essential
- The use of psychological, behavioural and physical interventions is recommended in addition to medication
- Patients and their families should receive information about pain
- Pain assessment and treatment should be conducted early to provide a foundation on which to build further constructive pain management interventions throughout a patient's life
- Cognitive therapies should be used to enhance coping strategies and reduce negative thoughts

Further reading

Dunlop R. and Bennett K. (2006) Pain management for sickle cell disease. *Cochrane Database of Systematic Reviews*, http://mrw.interscience.wiley.com/cochrane/clsysrev/articles/CD003350/pdf_fs.html.

Green A. (2002) Psychological therapies for sickle cell disease and pain. *Cochrane Database of Systematic Reviews*, http://mrw.interscience.wiley.com/cochrane/clsysrev/articles/CD001916/pdf_fs.html.

NHS (2006) *Sickle Cell Disease in Childhood: Standards and Guidelines*. NHS Sickle Cell and Thalassaemia Screen Programme in partnership with the Sickle Cell Society, http://www.sicklean-dthal.org.uk/Documents/DETAILED_CLIN_Oct19.pdf.

Mood disorder and pain

It is now well documented that most patients with chronic pain suffer from a number of co-morbid psychiatric conditions including depression, anxiety and personality disorders. The impact of these conditions on pain perception and recovery in acute pain is also gaining interest. However, there is always a danger that any psychiatric co-morbidity may be used as an excuse by healthcare professionals to explain pain that is confounding a diagnosis or organic explanation. As we gradually begin to unravel some of the intricacies of pain, psychology and psychiatry, it is already possible to identify some psychiatric disorders that may be involved in altering pain perception, such as:

- anxiety
- depression
- post-traumatic stress disorder
- hypochondriasis
- somatoform disorder
- Munchausen syndrome.

Anxiety

A relationship between anxiety and acute pain has been well established. Walsh (1993) studied pain and anxiety in an A&E department and reported the value of keeping patients informed. Anxiety may result in increased muscle tension that can ultimately lead to increased pain and fatigue. What has become apparent more recently is the impact of anxiety on chronic pain and especially the relationship of 'fear avoidance' and its negative impact on rehabilitation for patients with chronic musculoskeletal pain. Anxiety makes pain less tolerable, and anxiety about pain can become the major source of distress. 'Fear avoidance' refers to the fear of activity that may cause pain, particularly if this pain is then misinterpreted as a signal of further damage. Patients risk becoming deconditioned and losing confidence, and then they risk further disability as muscles weaken, ligaments and tendons tighten from loss of use and function becomes compromised.

Depression

Experiencing chronic pain would make anybody depressed, but in some instances it is difficult to establish exactly which came first: depression, leading an individual to become predisposed to pain, or pain causing the individual to become depressed about his or her situation. It has been suggested that some patients suffering chronic pain may overestimate the intensity of past painful episodes because the mood associated with their current pain is similar to the mood they experienced when they first had the pain. Depression associated with chronic pain may range from a temporary bad mood, a reaction to the current painful distress, to a chronic or major state of depression. Manchikanti et al. (2001) showed the presence of a major depressive disorder in 22% of a population with chronic pain compared to only 4% of the population without pain. Overall research suggests that depression in some form is experienced by 40–50% of chronic pain sufferers. Any attempts to improve pain control will be compromised unless we are aware of the impact of depression on patients. Fortunately, there are now some good assessment tools available that help to identify depression in patients with pain.

Post-traumatic stress disorder

We know stress can influence our response to pain. Being involved in an accident or incident, particularly if this may have been fatal, can impact negatively on pain recovery. This is particularly the case if the individual had no sense of control and felt emotionally overwhelmed. Loss of confidence may well be a big issue as well as reliving events, panic attacks, poor sleep quality and fear. Being aware of the events leading to the injury or trauma may assist a nurse or other healthcare professional to help a patient readjust, and gradually regain the confidence they need to rehabilitate effectively.

Case history

Georgina is a young woman of 20 who sustained a serious back injury after falling down a cliff. Although a ledge broke her fall, she could have fallen over 200 feet to her death. While walking with friends, they were larking about, when Georgina's shoes slipped on the wet grass. She initially fell over the top of the cliff but had managed to grab some vegetation to break her fall. She hung on for what seemed like ages with her friends desperately trying to reach her hand. Although rescue had been called, she reached a point when she could hang on no longer and the vegetation was gradually giving way. As she fell, she was convinced that she would die as she crashed on the rocks below. She was being treated for her injuries and her pain but her slow recovery was causing concern. Nobody was aware of the exact circumstances of her injury or the terror she had experienced in those minutes before she let go of the vegetation. Skilled counselling helped her to face her fears and understand how this was impacting on her recovery.

Hypochondriasis

This condition has been described as an overawareness of bodily sensations leading to an apprehension of disease and phobic concern. Patients may become fixated on the fear of having a life-threatening medical condition. It is suggested that this term is overused and obsolete, too often being used by clinicians when pain proves difficult to explain. However, we need to be aware that this condition may well be relevant, as the American Psychiatric Association (2000) has estimated the prevalence as 2–7% in the primary care outpatient setting.

Somatoform disorders

Somatoform disorders describe physical symptoms which present as pain in cutaneous and deeper tissues such as bone, ligaments and muscle. It is said to arise in late adolescence or the early twenties in patients who present with a history of multiple complaints, often occurring in clusters, for which no sufficient physical cause can be found (Tyrer 1992). The term seems to be used these days to describe what in the past was claimed to be hypochondriasis. Assessment for atypical masked depression should be included in the differential diagnosis in elderly patients with somatic complaints and multidisciplinary management is recommended, with the inclusion of a psychiatrist. Oyama (2007) contains a useful overview of somatoform disorders.

Munchausen syndrome

This is a complex psychological problem that is also described as a somatoform disorder. Patients may present with dramatic presentations of illness, which have been deliberately induced. They may fake symptoms and falsify investigations in order to obtain care. Patients with this disorder may go to extreme lengths in order to enter the 'sick role' such as swallowing razor blades, taking medications or adding blood to urine or other specimens. Pain may be part of the picture but not always. For a more in-depth explanation of this complex syndrome, see eMedicine (2006).

Case history

Mary Jones has been admitted to the female surgical ward with low abdominal pain, increasing in intensity to 8/10 over the 24 hours prior to her admission. Mary is 42 years old and lives with her husband and only child in a small town 100 miles away – they had been staying locally with her sister when the pain started. Over the next 48 hours numerous investigations were carried out, the results all being negative. Although kept nil by mouth in case of surgery and using a PCA pump for pain relief, Mary seemed content with the situation. It was decided that a decision would be made on the Wednesday doctors' round when Professor Richards was available. Meanwhile, a large set of notes arrived from her local hospital, cataloguing a series of similar painful episodes over the past 10 years, which had resulted in numerous surgical investigations. All had drawn a blank as nothing abnormal could be found.

During the Wednesday round, Professor Richards sat down with Mary and her husband and explained as gently as he could that surgery was unlikely to help her pain and that he was not prepared to operate. This news was met with extreme anger and tears from Mary, but this gradually gave way to a different emotion. As Professor Richards explained that he would not operate because it would not get rid of her pain, he said he wanted to give her a real chance of getting better and would refer her to someone who would help her with her pain and the havoc it was wreaking on her life. A referral was made to a clinical psychologist, and although the expectations were that Mary would be angry, she was not. That evening she seemed happier and her pain had diminished. Someone had confronted her and realised that she was unhappy. Recognising this and being strong enough to talk openly about this with her meant that at last she had the prospect of a new start.

Summary

Disordered thought, perception and behaviour are a relatively new field of study for the pain specialist, and, as stated previously, there is always a danger that when pain cannot be explained easily by the presence of obvious pathological factors, it will automatically be dismissed as being psychological in origin. As we start to understand the complex neurophysiology of pain, there is a risk in thinking that we may have the answers but as soon as we begin to gain some understanding, the more complex it becomes. For chronic pain, an endless search for a definite diagnosis or physical cause can lead to years of frustration, anger and pain. Modern technology does not always have the answers, so it is better to focus on helping someone to live with their pain through effective coping strategies than to search fruitlessly to find out 'why'. When the cause cannot be treated, helping sufferers live with and come to terms with their pain must always be the goal.

Further reading

Crofford L. (2007) Violence, stress and somatic syndromes. *Trauma, Violence and Abuse*, **8**(3): 299–313.

Lepine J., Zajecka J. and Krishnan R. (2007) *Mood Disorders: Management and Treatment Strategies for the 21st Century*. Three lectures available via Medscape, Lepine J., Depression and the body: diagnosing and treating depressed patients who present with somatic symptoms; Krishnan R., Depression and comorbid anxiety: evaluation and treatment for better outcomes; Kajecka J., Recognizing and managing treatment resistant depression, http://www.medscape.com/viewarticle/549528.

NHS Direct, Munchausen syndrome, http://cks.library.nhs.uk/patient_information_leaflet/munchausens_syndrome/introduction.

Substance misuse

Pain experienced by patients with a history of substance misuse

> There are few clinical situations more challenging, frustrating or stressful than the management of acute or chronic pain in patients known or suspected to be misusers [of chemicals]. (Payne 1989, p. 46)

How true this statement is to anyone who has ever managed the care of a patient in pain with a history of opioid use for recreation rather than pain relief. In the past, society has tended to blame patients for their own inadequacies (Stimmel 1989), but as we are coming to understand more about the dual problems of relieving pain and the complexities of addiction, we are faced with a need to know more about the management of these complicated and challenging patients.

We endeavoured to clarify some of the misconceptions surrounding the terminology associated with substance misuse in Chapter 4. To recap:

- *Substance misuse* exists when the extent and pattern of substance use interferes with the psychological and sociocultural integrity of the person. For example, there may be recurring problems with social and personal interactions or with the legal system, recurrent failures to fulfil work or family obligations, or patients may find themselves in physically hazardous situations (for example driving a car while under the influence of the substance), also putting others at risk (American Psychiatric Association 1994).

- *Physical dependence* occurs when a patient manifests symptoms of withdrawal when a drug is suddenly stopped – *it is not a sign that a patient is addicted but merely that the patient's body has become dependent on a substance*, often one that mimics an endogenous substance. The sudden withdrawal of this substance can lead to unpleasant side effects while the body tries to adjust. Although withdrawal symptoms – or 'cold turkey' as it is referred to among addicts and laypeople – are often associated with 'drug addiction', non-addicted patients may exhibit the same symptoms. For these patients, the symptoms can always be avoided if the drugs are withdrawn slowly rather than suddenly halted over night.

- *Tolerance* is defined as the need to administer larger doses of a drug in order to obtain the same effect. It usually occurs after repeated doses of opioid-based drugs. Again, it is not a sign of addiction but one of the body becoming 'used' to a drug. In the case of cancer patients, it can often signal an increase in pathology, or disease progression.

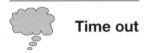 **Time out**

How often in your clinical area do you hear staff and patients voice concerns regarding addiction? Are their concerns justified? How many patients have a real addiction? If you have looked after someone with addiction who has pain, was their pain recognised and adequately controlled?

It is quite probable that these patients did not have their pain properly recognised and assessed. Have you ever seen 'avoid. opioids' written on the drug charts of patients admitted to hospital in pain who happen to be heroin addicts? Hopefully, with the clinical guidelines currently available, this scenario is rare but there are still incidences where a patient's pain has not been controlled adequately, and they are left to suffer withdrawal symptoms that cause additional pain and distress. When painful trauma or disease is present, it is not the time to make judgements or attempt to get a patient 'off drugs'. In fact, additional opioids will be necessary, often in very large quantities to overcome tolerance, counter withdrawal and provide analgesia.

Withdrawal is unpleasant and can be completely avoided, provided that opioids are not stopped rapidly. The symptoms are easy to identify:

- hypertension
- tachycardia

- abdominal pain
- muscle aches
- yawning
- diarrhoea
- rhinorrhea
- lacrimation
- vomiting and diarrhoea
- goose pimples.

Managing pain control in the opioid-abusing patient

In the management of pain in opioid-abusing patients, you should set realistic goals, explaining that, although you will endeavour to control their pain as effectively as possible, because of acquired tolerance, the control of their pain will be more difficult to achieve. These patients often accept this and in fact expect this to be the case. They can often be disarmingly grateful that anybody is taking the time and effort to recognise and try to alleviate their pain. Many will have had poor past experiences of healthcare facilities. The very nature of their lifestyle means that they have often experienced severe pain in the past, as well as being prone to trauma, infection, abscess formation and general ill health. It might have been their experience on previous hospital admissions to have their pain ignored, their addiction being seen as their own fault.

We cannot underestimate the frustration and negative feelings that many health-care professionals experience when having to nurse profoundly ill patients on a busy ward whose condition is a result of self-abuse such as opioid or alcohol addiction. It is all too easy to be judgmental, but we often have no insight into the sort of background that many of these people have endured. Sometimes all they have known is a life on the street; they may present as personally neglected, abusive and difficult. That is, however, probably the only life they know, often coming from an environment that is harsh and dangerous. The only language they are familiar with is abusive and crude. We know from the literature that some clinicians will hold negative views of these patients. Corley and Goren (1998) found that nurse behaviours often mirror the predominant values of society. One of the nurses from a focus group stated: 'The nursing profession is a very rule-laden profession and you're dealing with your ultimate rule breakers [substance misusers].'

Attempting to manage these patients' pain can, however, offer great reward. Patience and collaboration will frequently lead to the development of a therapeutic relationship that does not have to be negative for staff. We would not presume that the development of this therapeutic relationship is going to be easy; it has to be one of negotiation, trust and teamwork.

The assessment of pain will present special challenges. Although pain rating methods are always subjective, subjectivity is even more apparent in the patient with a history of opioid misuse. A very high pain score will almost always be the norm, but assessment is still necessary for a long-term comparison to evaluate different treatments. Differentiating between a high pain score and drug-seeking pain behaviour can sometimes prove impossible. While a patient is receiving active treatment for a potentially painful medical condition is not the time to disbelieve or question high pain scores. Nobody likes to be duped by a patient, but as there is no way of verifying patient reports of severe pain, we have no real alternative but to accept what they say.

While patients are in the healthcare system, we have a duty to recognise their pain and do our best to alleviate it, even though in some instances we may suspect that we are being used to fuel a habit. However, denying adequate treatment usually means that the patient will self-discharge or get his or her friends to bring in supplies. This can be dangerous if you do not know how much, or with what, patients are topping up their analgesia. There is also the dilemma of what to do if you suspect that a patient has a locker full of street heroin. Do you breach trust and search the locker, call the police, confront the patient? It is surely much better to foster an open and honest relationship from the start and work collaboratively with the patient; remember too that they will probably know far more about most of these drugs than you do.

Case history

Jane Wilson is a 21-year-old who has been working for six years as a prostitute to fuel a heroin addiction she has had since a boyfriend introduced her to the drug when she was just 14. In a desperate bid to end her life, or more probably in a desperate plea for help, she has taken an overdose of sleeping tablets and jumped out of a second-storey window, landing on the grass below. She is unconscious when her friends find her three hours later. They think that she has just had a 'bad trip' and drag her upstairs to bed. The following morning, Jane is conscious and tells her friends she has a terrible pain in her heels, ankles and knees, and that her back hurts. The pain is so bad that she begs her friends to give her a shot of heroin before calling the ambulance. When the paramedics arrive, they are unsure of what has happened or the extent of Jane's injuries. She is difficult to rouse, but when she is finally roused, she is abusive and uncooperative.

Jane is taken to A&E with a history obtained from her friends that she has taken a drug, has had a bad trip and has fallen over. It is almost impossible to obtain a history from Jane, but the department staff suspect that Jane has been a substance misuser for some time as she has needle marks up both her arms. As a result, she needs a central line in her neck in order for them to obtain intravenous access. Because Jane is so difficult to obtain a history from and her friends have been unable to help much, she is given some naloxone to reverse the heroin. She becomes almost impossible to manage, but numerous X-rays enable A&E staff to confirm that Jane has multiple fractures of her legs, a fracture of her pelvis and a non-displaced fracture of her lower spine.

Although Jane is given some additional opioid pain relief once the naloxone has worn off, the amount is not sufficient to counteract the symptoms of opioid with-drawal that develop quite rapidly. For the next 36 hours, over a weekend, Jane receives totally inadequate analgesia. Threatening to discharge herself from hospital, she is finally seen by the acute pain team in an extremely distressed state. Her pain is described as unbearable, and she is in acute withdrawal.

This case history may seem extreme, but in the authors' experience, it is not that uncommon.

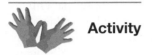 **Activity**

If you get the opportunity to talk to a patient with a history of opioid misuse, ask them how they would like to have pain managed while they are in hospital. Many have had such bad previous experiences that they are delighted when somebody takes the trouble to obtain information from their perspective.

More recently, hospitals and clinical care teams will have agreed guidelines or a protocol, which can make effective pain management a more achievable goal.

Key points for effective care of patients with opioid dependency should include the following:

- If you suspect that a patient may be misusing substances, try to confirm this as early as possible. Many will be quite honest and open about their addiction, especially if they know that you are trying to control their pain.
- Make sure you contact people with specialist knowledge; your acute pain team, pharmacist, local drug and alcohol advisory team, and palliative care teams may be able to help, especially 'out of hours', if you are encountering problems getting opioid dosages correct.
- Ensure that only one person is responsible for prescribing medication in order to avoid multiple changes and the prescription of incompatible drugs, for example a partial agonist or agonist/antagonist, as this could lead to withdrawal symptoms.
- Use PCA where practical and possible, remembering that the bolus dose often has to be at least twice or even three times the normal dose.
- Ensure that the patient receives sufficient opioids to control withdrawal and provide pain relief; the doses often have to be very high. Try to establish how much opioid the patient takes on a daily basis, but remember that this will only be a rough guide as street drugs can vary considerably in quality and strength, and some patients will be quite creative for fear that you will underestimate their need. Unfortunately, heroin has in the past few years become cheaper and easier to obtain so patients can often tolerate extremely high doses.
- Where possible, use combination therapy, that is, opioids, NSAIDS, local anaesthetics, adjuvants and non-pharmacological strategies.
- Collaborate with patients, obtaining their trust and setting realistic goals.
- Not only may you encounter patients who are substance misusers, but as we now use opioids more generally to treat chronic non-malignant pain, it is important to be aware of the predictors of opioid misuse. Studies so far suggest that this risk is higher in patients with a self-reported history of alcohol or cocaine misuse or previous criminal convictions for drug offences.

See the British Pain Society's (2005) recommendations for the appropriate use of opioids for persistent non-cancer pain.

Before we leave the topic of substance misuse and addiction, it is worth reminding readers that undertreating pain because of fear of addiction predisposes patients to the development of pseudo-addictive behaviour. This is characterised by seeking and hoarding drugs, but in this case the behaviour is driven by a fear of pain, usually spurred on by inadequate pain management in the past. The behaviour usually disappears when pain is managed effectively. Healthcare professionals may label this drug-seeking behaviour and be highly suspicious but it could be described as more a pain avoidance behaviour than a sign of addiction. Proper pain assessment should help to reduce this problem (Australian and New Zealand College of Anaesthetists and Faculty of Pain Medicine 2005).

Intractable pain and secondary gain/loss

'Intractable' is a term often used when, despite everyone's best efforts, a patient's pain remains stubbornly resistant to any sort of influence, therapy or cure. Although currently not well defined, the term 'secondary gain' has been used to describe the possible influence that practical, financial or emotional advantage may have on pain becoming intractable. In instances where a person may gain some advantage from his or her pain, breaking the cycle of pain and pain behaviour can become extremely difficult.

These patients are not malingering, which is described as lying about the existence of pain, and is said to be quite rare (McCaffery and Beebe 1994). What appears to happen is that an initial trauma or disease, which may have been very painful at the time, results in ongoing pain way beyond the time the pain would have been expected to subside. The pain is very real but in this instance could be linked more to psychosocial issues such as the solicitous attention of others, particularly family, and temporary relief from responsibilities. This is usually combined with feelings of distress, poor coping strategies, loss of self-esteem and social isolation, driving a complex interplay between mind and body. Studies have been undertaken on secondary gain in the form of compensation payments and involvement in legal action. However, data so far have suggested that compensation has a minor role in explaining anything about ongoing pain (Rohling et al. 1995). More work is now being undertaken on the impact of secondary loss and the equally large barrier to effective treatment this can have on patients in pain. Personal losses can include the economic consequences of losing a job and the social relationships and support network that a working environment can offer. There is also the issue of social stigma and guilt associated with 'disability' as well as the loss of recreational activities and the respect of friends and family (Fishbain 1994).

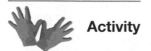 **Activity**

Do you know a friend, relative or patient who is 'disabled' with intractable pain, which causes them a great deal of suffering and distress? Now make a short list of factors that may inhibit strategies to improve how such individuals cope with their pain. Could subtle factors be contributing to their failure to come to terms with their pain and adapt their lives to it? What enables some individuals to live with pain but still enjoy quality of life while others become deeply unhappy, socially isolated and totally overwhelmed?

The following are normally regarded as the 'secondary gain' drivers of pain disability:

- attention from healthcare professionals
- attention from friends and family
- sanctioned avoidance of stress at work
- sanctioned avoidance of domestic role
- reduced responsibility
- loss of feelings of control
- outstanding litigation
- being in receipt of disability living allowance (DLA) or incapacity benefit.

Dissatisfaction with healthcare professionals may develop as multiple encounters fail to be effective. This inevitably leads to tension, anger, conflict and possibly hostility. Without a proper explanation for their continuing pain, individuals can become increasingly inactive as they associate 'undiagnosed' pain with further damage. They often increase their analgesic drug use, which has a further negative effect on mood and activity. Inactivity leads to disability and exhaustion and fatigue take over. Patients withdraw from activities and social interactions that used to give them pleasure, focusing more and more on their pain. Dependency sets in, and resentment may spread. When illness behaviour eventually fails to elicit a benevolent response, conflict extends further to friends and family.

Social policy

It could be argued that we now live within a social infrastructure that may be seen to support dependency rather than the positive strategies that encourage sufferers to return to as normal a life as possible. It is worthwhile considering the vast amount of money being paid in DLA, incapacity benefit and so on compared with the tiny fraction of the chancellor's coffers that is spent on pain management, rehabilitation facilities and back to work initiatives. However, in light of recent government initiatives and the Green Paper *No one Written off: Reforming Welfare to Reward Responsibility* (DWP 2008), this might be gradually changing. Consider also the fact that we now have aggressive health and safety policies within the workplace, with a steep decline in the number of heavy and hazardous industries such as coal mining. Between 1986 and 1992, however, the figure for incapacity benefit being paid for back pain rose by 104%, and until recently was rising annually. This is coupled with the fact that there is no evidence of an increasing frequency of physical trauma or other organic cause (Potter 1998). It would appear that something is very amiss indeed with the social infrastructures of Western societies.

The influence of litigation

There has now been extensive work on the possible influence that adversarial compensation litigation might have on the long-term outcome following an acute injury. Previously a common view was that financial secondary gain could be equated with conscious malingering and that if patients are being paid to be sick, they will learn to continue those behaviours that reward them (Hammonds et al. 1978). However, researchers have not confirmed these assumptions but have found that while exaggerated self-reported physical symptoms are more extreme when financial secondary gain exists, resolution of financial claims does not necessarily resolve the perceived dysfunction or disability (Evans 1992).

In most Western societies, even in the presence of pain, government and clinicians are now advocating the need to advise patients to return to work much earlier than was normal in the 1980s and 90s. Although this invariably meets with an angry response, it is argued that this approach is an important part of overall treatment for patients with chronic pain receiving workers' compensation or incapacity benefit. The importance of early intervention is vital for those who cease working; the passage of inactive time can hinder rather than heal. Statistics show that once someone has been on incapacity benefit for one year, they are likely to be there for eight. And once they've been on it for two years, they are more likely to die or retire as an incapacity benefit recipient than they are ever to work again (Johnson 2004).

Patients with chronic musculoskeletal pain could well be engaged in less effective coping styles, feel less in control and display extremely compromised physical functioning.

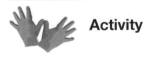 **Activity**

Have you looked after a patient who was receiving, or attempting to claim, compensation following some work-related injury? What sort of job did he or she have: was it absorbing and interesting, or was it boring and repetitive?

Relief from responsibility, poor job satisfaction and high mental stress

Recent evidence also suggests that psychosocial factors, particularly for conditions such as low back pain, have an influence as great, if not greater, on disability as on ergonomic aspects (Symonds et al. 1996). A job that is perceived as unrewarding and repetitive may significantly impact on an individual's desire to continue with that work. Anger is also commonly observed in patients with chronic pain and this may be directed towards an employer or the workplace if an injury was sustained at work. This may be combined with frustration at the persistence of symptoms and treatment failures, the response of insurance companies and healthcare practitioners if difficulties are encountered while trying to receive appropriate treatment (Gatchel 2004). Feelings of internalised anger have been strongly related to measures of pain intensity, pain behaviour and perceived interference with activities of daily living (Kerns et al. 1994).

The influence of the family

Family, friends and carers may unwittingly play a part in perpetuating disability. When we are ill, especially when we are admitted to hospital, we receive cards, flowers and the solicitous visits of friends and family. Other family members take over chores and relieve us of day-to-day household responsibilities.

For most people, this becomes self-limiting as the acute phase of an illness diminishes, but if chronic pain causes a patient's role to become far more passive and dependent, the altered family dynamics may unwittingly contribute to further disability as family members gradually take over the patient's role. If positive strategies to achieve improved mobility and reinforce 'well' behaviour are not fully understood by the family, rehabilitation programmes can be doomed to failure.

Case history

Mrs Bain is a 56-year-old woman with two daughters in their twenties and a son aged 17. Some years ago, she hurt her back lifting a box at work. She has been left with chronic back pain, which she has been told is the result of a 'slipped disc' and general degeneration of her spine. Mrs Bain also has mild osteoporosis for which she is now taking hormone replacement therapy. She has become very bitter at the medical profession's seeming inability to do anything to help her pain. She is also angry that the injury occurred at work as she felt she shouldn't have been placed in a situation where a box needed to be moved in the first place.

Despite being advised against surgery by her GP and physiotherapist, Mrs Bain has had spinal fusion surgery. Prior to surgery, she had been given two epidural injections, one of which had reduced her pain for at least six weeks. With the failure of surgery, she now demands and receives regular caudal epidural injections with little or no benefit. She has been admitted to hospital many times for no active treatment other than pain relief, which never really works. She is frequently taken to A&E, and the family call out their GP on a regular basis. Nothing ever satisfactorily controls Mrs Bain's pain and she now spends most of her time either in bed or lying on the sofa. She feels that all her pain is related to 'damage' to her spine and if she does too much she will only make it worse – especially as her 'bones are fragile' as a result of her osteoporosis. Her family are extremely supportive and concerned, undertaking all the domestic chores between them. Mrs Bain now rarely goes out, but if she does, she uses a wheelchair. She is very depressed, cries frequently, has gained considerable weight and no longer sees her friends. Her family are at their wits' end.

Partial solution:
Although Mrs Bain's story represents a common but challenging case that you may encounter in either primary or secondary care, some solutions can be helpful.

Mrs Bain is finally admitted onto a rehabilitation programme that aims to reduce her dependency on analgesia, improve her mood and quality of life and increase her mobility. She undergoes an extensive assessment that includes a comprehensive physical examination alongside assessment for the psychosocial impact of her pain. She shows signs of clinical depression and is prescribed an antidepressant. Four weeks later she started on a six-week programme that sets goals on a daily basis in terms of performing tasks and extending her range and scope of mobility, thereby eliminating the need to use aids such as the wheelchair. Mrs Bain's husband is included in all the patient education components of the programme, and the entire family are urged to substitute 'doing everything' with supporting and encouraging Mrs Bain to do more for herself. Group sessions and specific input from an experienced clinical psychologist help Mrs Bain to come to terms with her anger and bitterness. She gradually starts to accept some personal responsibility for her situation and the poor outcome from what initially was a rather trivial 'injury'.

Such programmes can be very successful in improving patient self-confidence and mobility, thereby reducing disability. They never claim to be able to remove pain, but as patients become more socially interactive, physically fitter and more confident in their ability to cope with their pain, often their quality of life improves. In some cases, it has been reported that the pain has spontaneously resolved.

Further reading

Johnson A. (2004) Pathways to work: enabling rehabilitation. Speech by the secretary of state for work and pensions to the Royal Society of Medicine, 12 October, http://www.dwp.gov.uk/aboutus/2004/18_10_04_prrsm.asp.
DWP (Department of Work and Pensions) (2008) *No one Written off: Reforming Welfare to Reward Responsibility*, http://www.dwp.gov.uk/welfarereform/noonewrittenoff/noonewrittenoff-complete.pdf

Conclusion

In this chapter, we have discussed the importance of considering other factors, apart from an original pathological cause, that can impact on a person's experience of pain. Building on the previous chapters, we have explored a more complex picture, where the nature of pain is compounded by numerous other factors, often interrelated. It is this complexity that frequently challenges those providing pain relief. In addition to the physiological cause of pain, it is the overlapping layers such as cultural background, family life, work and depression that create the tapestry of complexity. We have briefly introduced some theories that help to describe how pain sufferers explain or come to terms with the origins of their pain and the extent to which they are prepared to take responsibility for it. The management of pain for these people will always be challenging but knowledge and understanding can work well to create a strong platform upon which to build individualised pain care.

After a break, try the multiple choice test below in order to self-assess your learning so far. For some of the questions more than one answer will be correct, however, there will be one answer that is so far best supported by the evidence.

Nursing Patients with Challenging Pain
Multiple choice TEST

1. On what does the degree of suffering from burn pain depend?
   a. The age of the person, as young children feel less pain due to immature neural networks ☐
   b. The pain tolerance of an individual ☐
   c. The depth of tissue damage ☐
   d. It cannot be predicted ☐

2. When assessing pain in patients suffering an acute sickle-cell crisis, which is likely to be the best approach?
   a. Ask patients to rate their pain intensity on a numerical or verbal rating scale ☐
   b. Watch for elevations in blood pressure or pulse rate ☐
   c. Ask patients about their pain and use a rating scale to assess its intensity ☐
   d. Avoid encouraging patients to focus on their pain but observe them for pain behaviours ☐

3. Which of the following therapies have patients with spinal cord injury reported most consistently as helpful?
   a. Guided imagery ☐
   b. Cold therapy ☐
   c. Massage ☐
   d. Reflexology ☐

4. Which of the following people are most at risk of sickle-cell disease?
   a. Caucasians ☐
   b. Asians ☐
   c. Latin Americans ☐
   d. African/Caribbeans ☐

5. When does sickle-cell disease manifest itself and pain become a problem?
   a. In infancy ☐
   b. In childhood ☐
   c. In adolescence ☐
   d. In adults ☐

6. Depression is a common experience for people with chronic pain but what does research so far suggest is the incidence of a major depressive disorder in patients with chronic pain?
   a. 5% ☐
   b. 17% ☐
   c. 22% ☐
   d. 40% ☐

7. Which one of the following opioid drugs could cause withdrawal symptoms in a patient addicted to heroin?
   a. Oxycontin ☐
   b. Buprenorphine ☐
   c. Morphine ☐
   d. Fentanyl ☐

8. Which of the following is not normally associated with opioid withdrawal syndrome?
   a. Yawning ☐
   b. Watery eyes ☐
   c. Hypotension ☐
   d. Runny nose ☐

9. You have a heroin addict admitted to your ward who has also just undergone surgery to remove his spleen. Which of the following goals do you feel is the most important to achieve during his admission to hospital?
   a. A gradual reduction in opioid dependency ☐
   b. Adequate analgesia involving large doses of opioids ☐
   c. Enrolling the patient onto a drug rehabilitation programme ☐
   d. Trying to avoiding opioids altogether by treating the pain with NSAIDs and adjuvant medication ☐

10. What is a somatoform disorder?
    a. A complaint of pain in large joints ☐
    b. A complaint of pain over certain anatomical 'trigger' points ☐
    c. A complaint of generalised abdominal pain ☐
    d. A complaint of multiple sites of pain with no obvious connection or physical cause ☐

Answers

1. d. It cannot be predicted; burns may include a mixture of deep burns (tending to give less pain because of nerve endings being damaged) and superficial burns (often very painful). The age of the person is not significant. Young children may need greater reassurance and comfort, as they might not be able to respond verbally to pain assessment. All patients who have been burnt will feel pain. The expression of that pain and its meaning for an individual will vary depending on a person's tolerance to pain; although many other factors will affect their suffering.

2. c. Ask patients about their pain and use a rating scale to assess its intensity; this is the best answer as this approach immediately confirms to patients that you are interested in their pain. The rating of pain intensity supplements the data you have collected and can be useful to evaluate the effectiveness of any interventions. With an acute exacerbation of a chronic disease, it is unlikely that a simple pain intensity rating such as the 0–10 scale will tell you very much about the pain other than intensity. It will not give you location, quality or impact of the pain. Similarly, with someone who has experienced chronic pain, it is unlikely that physiological parameters will be accurate in reflecting that pain, as these may remain 'normal'. Severe pain can sometimes cause 'shock', the blood pressure and pulse rate falling, but for pain assessment, these are unreliable measures and are best avoided as they can lead to inaccurate conclusions. Encouraging someone to focus on their chronic pain can reduce the effectiveness of distraction strategies; however, during a painful crisis, pain can be very severe and will need regularly assessing to establish analgesia.

3. c. In research so far, most patients have rated massage as the most helpful non-pharmacological therapy. There is little research available on spinal cord injury and guided imagery or reflexology, although heat therapy has been rated as effective in some groups. Cold therapy is usually unpopular for the treatment of chronic pain.

4. d. African/Caribbeans; the condition is most common in this group and is caused by a genetic mutation passed on through certain families.

5. a. In infancy; individuals are born with the condition, which is currently incurable.

6. c. 22% of patients with chronic pain have shown symptoms of a major depressive disorder. Overall, some form of depression is reported to be as high as 40–100% of patients with chronic pain in various studies. Given the nature of the pain, it is perhaps unsurprising that depression is such a major feature.

7. b. Buprenorphine, as it is a partial opioid angonist. This means that it can, in theory, partially block the action of a pure agonist such as the three others which are all mu receptor agonists.

8. c. Hypotension is not normally associated with withdrawal syndrome, although hypertension and an increase in pulse rate can sometimes be seen as a reaction to the stress and anxiety caused by acute withdrawal. Yawning, watery eyes and a runny nose are very common symptoms of withdrawal and will often be a valuable clue, should a patient be denying withdrawal or staff be unfamiliar with the symptoms.

9. b. Adequate analgesia involving large doses of opioids is the most appropriate answer. Although a gradual reduction in opioid dependency and enrolling a patient on a drug rehabilitation programme are commendable goals to aim for, it is highly unlikely these will

be successful once a patient is in hospital and experiencing pain and stress away from his or her usual support strategies; it is probably inappropriate to articulate these goals during the acute phase of the patient's recovery. Treating the pain with NSAIDs alone would almost certainly lead to the patient experiencing painful and distressing withdrawal symptoms.

10. d. Somatoform disorder, although thought to be relatively rare, is usually associated with multiple sites of pain that can't be traced to a specific physical cause and medical tests are either normal or don't explain the symptoms. Although joint pain may a symptom, the complaint may also be whole limb pain rather than just specific joints. Anatomical 'trigger' points are usually associated with a condition termed 'fibromyalgia'. Again abdominal pain may be a feature but usually complaints involve at least two or more unexplained gastrointestinal symptoms such as nausea and indigestion as well as pain.

Glossary

Acute pain	Pain of recent onset and probable limited duration. It usually has an identifiable temporal and causal relationship to injury and disease (IASP, 1986)
Acute on chronic pain	An acutely painful flare-up of a chronic painful condition such as low back pain
Adjuvant therapy	Drugs that do not have an obvious analgesic action but can, because of the complex origins of some types of pain, provide relief in certain conditions and circumstances
Affective	The emotion and feelings generated by pain
Acquired immunodeficiency syndrome (AIDS)	The symptoms and infections resulting from damage to the immune system caused by the human immuno-deficiency virus (HIV)
Allodynia	A painful response to a normally non-painful stimuli like simple touch and is a feature of nerve damage
Angina	A painful tightness in the chest due to lack of blood and oxygen to the heart muscle
Aortic aneurysm	A bulge or weakness in the wall of the aorta
Atelectasis	Collapse of part or the entire lung
Autonomic	Part of the nervous system that helps to maintain homeostasis in the body regulating heart rate, digestion, respiratory rate and so on
Biliary disease	Inflammation, infection, stones or obstruction that affects the gall bladder
Biofeedback	A complementary therapy that encourages patients to become aware of bodily functions such as blood pressure, heart rate and muscle tension. With awareness of these functions, patients are coached to take more conscious control of these physiological activities
Bony metastasis	Cancer that has spread to the bones
Bradykinin	A peptide thought to have a role in the inflammatory process and maintenance of pain
Carpel tunnel syndrome	A disorder of the wrist, usually associated with a repetitive strain, that leads to compression of the median nerve to the hand and results in numbness and tingling

Catecholamines	A group of compounds produced by the body that play an important role in the body's response to stress, for example adrenaline and noradrenaline
Ceiling effect	Situation where increasing the dosage of a drug fails to produce more pain relief
Cholecystitis	A painful condition when there is blockage or infection of the gall bladder
Chronic pain	Pain lasting for a long period of time. It usually persists beyond the time of healing of an injury, and there is frequently no identifiable cause (IASP, 1986)
Chronic non-malignant or persistent pain	Ongoing pain not associated with malignant disease such as cancer
Chronic malignant pain	Pain associated with a life-limiting disease such as cancer
Diverticular disease	A common condition affecting the digestive system that occurs when bulges or pouches form in the wall of the bowel
Cortex of the brain	The cerebral cortex that forms the outer part of the brain and is associated with memory, attention, perceptual awareness, thought, language and consciousness
Cognitive	The thought processes that lead to knowledge, for example perception and reasoning
Complex regional pain syndrome	Also referred to as 'causalgia' or 'reflex sympathetic dystrophy'; is thought to be caused by injury to a peripheral nerve that results in severe pain, burning sensation, altered skin colour and texture
Cortisol	A hormone produced by the adrenal glands in response to stress
Cyclo-oxygenase (COX)	An enzyme responsible for the formation of prostaglandins, prostacyclin and thromboxane. The formation of prostaglandin E is associated with inflammatory pain
Cystic fibrosis (CF)	A hereditary condition that affects the glands of the lungs, liver and other organs, ultimately leading to multisystem failure
Deconditioning	Loss of physical fitness through illness or lack of exercise
Decompression sickness	Commonly termed the 'bends'; caused by nitrogen bubbles forming in the bloodstream and body tissues. It is usually associated with returning to the surface too rapidly following a dive in the sea

Dorsal horn of the spinal cord	Can be seen in a cross-section of the spinal cord and is composed of grey matter
Deep vein thrombosis (DVT)	The formation of a blood clot most commonly in the leg or pelvic veins
Endocrine	The system of organs that release hormones
Endogenous	A substance produced or synthesised within the body
Endorphin	One of a group of neuropeptides produced naturally by the body that reduce the perception of pain
Giant cell arteritis	Also termed 'temporal arteritis'; causes inflammation of the temporal arteries and may lead to blindness
Gout	A form of acute and painful arthritis, which can particularly affect the big toe and is associated with high levels of uric acid in the blood
Human immunodeficiency virus (HIV)	A retrovirus that attacks the immune system and can lead to acquired immunodeficiency syndromes (AIDS)
Hypoxemia	Reduction of oxygen in the blood
Hypoxia	A lack of oxygen
Iatrogenic	Complications or disease in a patient caused by physicians or treatment from a healthcare professional
Immune response	The mechanism that protects against disease by identifying and destroying pathogens and tumour cells
Immunosupression	The reduction of activity or efficacy of the immune system
Intermittent claudication	The cramping pain classically felt in the calf muscles during exercise and most commonly due to peripheral vascular disease
Intermittent pain	Pain that occurs occasionally or at regular, or irregular, intervals
Intractable pain	Pain that is not relieved in clinical practice despite all efforts. A term not often used these days
Intrathecal	The area under the arachnoid membrane covering the spinal cord and brain
Ischaemia	A restriction in the blood supply
Laminae	A layer or plate
Leukotriene	Produced by the body and thought to be responsible for the inflammatory response
Limbic	The system in the brain associated with emotion

Locus of control	A belief about whether we feel we can control outcomes by our thoughts and actions (internal) or whether we believe outcomes are outside our personal control (external)
Lymphoedema	Swelling of tissue as a result of an obstruction in the lymphatic system
Multimodal	Also termed 'balanced analgesia'; refers to the practice of combining two or more drugs and therapies to improve pain relief. Sometimes this practice enables drug doses to be reduced to lessen the risk of side effects while capitalising on the synergistic effect, for example combining paracetamol with an opioid
Multiple sclerosis	An autoimmune disease causing the immune system to gradually destroy the central nervous system
Myocardial infarction (MI)	Occurs when the blood supply to part of the heart is disrupted usually by a blood clot or plaque, commonly called a heart attack
Neuropathic pain	Usually regarded as a chronic pain associated with damage to or dysfunction of nerves. It may or may not be associated with actual tissue damage but is associated with trauma to nerves caused by injury or surgery, disease such as a virus, ischaemia, toxins or metabolic disorders such as diabetes
Neurosignature	A term devised by Melzack to describe a network of neurones in the brain that create impulses that inform the brain of one's own body and is prewired by genetics
Neurotransmitters	Chemicals that signal between nerve cells and to other cells in the body
Nerve block	The use of local anaesthetics onto or very close to a nerve to temporarily block the signal from that nerve. This can be permanent if nerve tissue is destroyed
NMDA (N-methyl-D-aspartic acid) receptors	Can become activated by prolonged firing of C fibres leading to spinal cord neurones becoming more responsive to subsequent input and less sensitive to opioids. The receptor is thought to be responsible for pain 'wind-up'
Nociceptive pain	The involvement of nociceptors – nerves that transmit pain following damage to tissue. They can be activated by tissue irritation, impending or actual injury transmitting signals from the periphery to the central nervous system

Noradrenaline	Released by the adrenal glands and prepares the body for the fight-or-flight response by increasing heart rate and blood pressure
Opioid	Generic term for all substances, both natural and synthetic, with a pharmacological action similar to morphine
Opioid receptors	The group of receptors found on nerves that are activated by opioids
Osteoarthritis	A degenerative joint disease caused by wearing of the cartilage that covers and cushions joints and the loss of synovial fluid
Osteoporosis	A disease that results in a decrease in bone mass and density, increasing the risk of fractures and bone deformities
Parasthesia	An abnormal sensation such as burning or prickling
Parkinson's disease	A degenerative disease that affects the central nervous system
Persistent pain	Pain that continues without interruption, being constant and unremitting
Persistent intermittent pain	Constant static pain with episodic flares that may occur in waves or patterns
Phantom pain	Pain felt to be coming from a limb or body part that has been amputated. The mechanism is not fully understood, but there are suggestions that it might arise from a peripheral origin in the severed nerves in response to changes in the brain or spinal cord
Plasticity	In terms of pain, describes the ability of nerves to alter and change. For example, if damage occurs in the brain, another area may take over some of the function
Pneumothorax	Air or gas in the pleural space that results in partial or complete lung collapse
Polymyalgia rheumatica	A painful condition experienced by older people
Postherpetic neuralgia	A nerve pain that persists after an attack of shingles
Post-stroke pain	Also referred to as 'thalamic pain syndrome'; is a neuropathic pain resulting from damage to the central nervous system usually following a stroke
Primary hyperalgesia	Increased pain sensation at the site of injury
Prophylactic	A medicine or treatment given to prevent a disease from occurring

Prostaglandins	Hormone-like substances that act on a wide range of body functions, particularly in the modulation of inflammation
Psychogenic	Disorders that originate in the mind rather than from an organic cause or pathology
Pulmonary embolism (PE)	A sudden blockage of a lung artery usually from a blood clot that has broken away from a deep vein thrombosis in the leg
Receptors	Proteins, usually located on cell membranes, that bind to specific molecules and initiate a cellular response
Referred pain	Pain that can arise when a visceral organ shares dorsal horn neurones transmitting sensation from the skin; this neurone may then cause the brain to incorrectly interpret the source of the pain
Reye's syndrome	A serious illness that can particularly affect the brain and liver and is associated with aspirin consumption in children
Secondary hyperalgesia	Increased pain sensation developing in tissue more distant from the site of injury
Serotonin	A hormone and neurotransmitter with multiple functions but is particularly associated with mood
Somatic pain	Pain experienced in the skin, body wall and musculoskeletal system
Somatosensory	Areas of the brain that process information from somatic receptors
Substance P	Involved in the transmission of information about tissue damage from the periphery to the central nervous system
Substantia gelatinosa	A dense area of neuronal tissue in the spinal cord vital for the reception and modulation of pain messages from the periphery
Syringomyelia	A disease of the spinal cord leading to the development of cavities in the cord, spasticity and sensory disturbance
Systemic lupus erythematosus (SLE)	An autoimmune disease where the immune system attacks cells and tissue resulting in inflammation and damage
Thalamus	An important 'relay' part of the brain involved in both processing and relaying sensory information to other parts of the brain. It has a complex role and is also thought to play a part in regulating arousal, levels of awareness and activity

Titrated	The process of gradually adjusting the dose of a drug until the desired effect is achieved or side effects make further adjustment unacceptable
Tractable pain	Pain that is controlled
Vagal tone	Impulses from the vagus nerve that control the resting heart beat
Venous leg ulcer	A skin sore in the lower leg due to the high pressure of blood in leg veins
Visceral pain	Pain in the internal organs
Wind-up	The process of increased central sensitisation of pain pathways in response to sustained input from nociceptors. It leads to increasing and spontaneous pain and allodynia
Wound dehiscence	A bursting or splitting of a wound. It is a complication of surgery where the wound does not heal properly

References

Abbey J., Piller N., DeBellis A., Esterman A., Parker D., et al. (2004) The Abbey Pain Scale. A 1 minute numerical indicator for people with late-stage dementia. *International Journal of Palliative Nursing*, **10**: 6–13.

Allcock N., Elkan R. and Williams J. (2007) Patients referred to a pain management clinic: beliefs, expectations and priorities. *Journal of Advanced Nursing*, **60**(3): 248–56.

Allison T., Symmons D., Brammah T, Haynes P., Rogers H. et al. (2002) Musculoskeletal pain is more generalised among people from ethnic minorities than among white people in Greater Manchester. *Annals of the Rheumatic Diseases*, **61**: 151–6.

Ambuel B., Hamlett K., Marx C. and Blumer J. (1992) Assessing distress in pediatric intensive care environments: The Comfort Scale. *Journal of Pediatric Psychology*, **17**: 95–109.

American Academy of Paediatrics and American Pain Society (2001) The assessment and management of acute pain in infants, children and adolescents. *Pediatrics*, **108**(3): 793–7.

American Geriatrics Society (2002) The management of persistent pain in older persons. *Journal of the American Geriatrics Society*, **50**(6): s205–24, http://www.americangeriatrics.org/products/positionpapers/JGS5071.pdf.

American Pain Society (APS) (1999) *Guidelines for the Management of Chronic Pain in Sickle Cell Disease*. Glenville, IL, APS.

American Psychiatric Association (1994) *Diagnostic and Statistical Manual of Mental Disorders*, 4th edn. Washington DC, American Psychiatric Association.

American Psychiatric Association (2000) *Diagnostic and Statistical Manual of Mental Disorders*, 4th edn rev. Washington DC, American Psychiatric Association.

Anand K. and the International Evidence-based Group for Neonatal Pain (2001) Consensus statement for the prevention and management of pain in the newborn. *Archives of Pediatrics & Adolescent Medicine*, **155**: 173–80.

Anand K. and Scalzo F. (2000) Can adverse neonatal experiences alter brain development and subsequent behaviour? *Biology of Neonate*, **77**: 69–72.

Anand K. and Maze M. (2001) Fetuses, fentanyl, and the stress response: signals from the beginnings of pain? *Anaesthesiology*, **95**: 823–5.

Apfelbaum J., Chen C., Mehta S. and Gan T. (2003) Postoperative pain experience: results from a national survey suggest postoperative pain continues to be undermanaged. *Anesthesia & Analgesia*, **97**: 534–40.

Assendelft W., Morton S., Yu El., Suttorp M. and Shekelle P. (2003) Spinal manipulative therapy for low back pain: a meta-analysis of effectiveness relative to other therapies. *Annals of Internal Medicine*, **138**: 871–81.

Astor R. (2001) Detecting pain in people with profound learning disabilities. *Nursing Times*, **97**(40): 38–9.

Australian and New Zealand College of Anaesthetists and Faculty of Pain Medicine (2005) *Acute Pain Management: Scientific Evidence*, 2nd edn, http://www.nhmrc.gov.au/publications/_files/cp104.pdf.

Backonja M. (2003) Defining neuropathic pain. *Anaesthesia & Analgesia*, **97**: 785–90.

Backonja M. and Serra J. (2004) Pharmacologic management Part 2: Lesser-studied neuropathic pain diseases. *Pain Medicine*, **5**(S1): S48–S59.

Ballantyne J.C., Carr D.B., Chalmers T.C., Dear K.G. and Angellilo I.F. (1993) Postoperative patient controlled analgesia: meta analyses of initial randomised controlled trials. *Journal of Clinical Anaesthesiology*, **5**: 182–93.

Bandolier (1997) Phytodolor for musculoskeletal pain, http://www.jr2.ox.ac.uk/bandolier/booth/alternat/AT026.html.

Bandolier (1999) Preoperative information-giving interventions and pain, http://www.jr2.ox.ac.uk/bandolier/booth/painpag/Acutrev/Other/AP061.html.

Bandolier (2002) Chronic pain after surgery, http://www.jr2.ox.ac.uk/bandolier/band103/b103-4.html.

Bandolier (2005) League table of analgesia, http://www.jr2.ox.ac.uk/bandolier/booth/painpag/acutrev/analgesics/leagtab.html.

Bell R., Dahl J., Moore R. and Kalso E. (2006) Perioperative ketamine for acute postoperative pain. *Cochrane Database of Systematic Reviews*, http://www.cochrane.org/reviews/en/ab004603.html.

Benjamin L., Swinson G. and Nagel R. (2000) Sickle cell anemia day hospital: an approach for the management of uncomplicated painful crises. *Blood*, **95**(4): 1130–6.

Bennett M., Smith B., Torrance N. and Potter J. (2003) The S-LANSS score for identifying pain of predominantly neuropathic origin: validation for use in clinical and postal research. *Journal of Pain*, **6**(3): 149–58.

Berwick D. (1998) Developing and testing changes in delivery of care. *Annals of Internal Medicine*, **128**(8): 651–6.

Bhutta A., Rovnaghi C., Simpson P., Gosset J., Scalzo F. et al. (2001) Interactions of inflammatory pain and morphine in infant rats: long-term behavioural effects. *Physiology & Behavior*, **73**: 51–8.

Bissell P., Ward P.R. and Noyce P.R. (2001) The dependent consumer: reflections on accounts of the risks of non-prescriptions medicines. *Health*, **5**(1): 5–30.

Blauer T. and Gertsmann D. (1998) A simultaneous comparison of three neonatal pain scales during common NICU procedures. *Clinical Journal of Pain*, **14**: 39–47.

Blomquist K and Edberg A. (2002) Living with persistent pain: experiences of older people receiving home care'. *Journal of Advanced Nursing*, **40**(3): 297–306.

Bodfish J., Harper V., Deacon J. and Symons F. (2001) Identifying and measuring pain in persons with developmental disabilities: a manual for the Pain and Discomfort Scale (PADS). Unpublished MS, Western Carolina Center, Morganton, NC.

Booker M., Blethyn K. and Wright C. (2006) Pain management in sickle cell disease. *Chronic Illness*, **2**(1): 39–50.

Booth K., Maguire P., Butterworth T. and Hillier V. (1996), Perceived professional support and the use of blocking behaviours by hospice nurses. *Journal of Advanced Nursing*, **24**(3): 522–7.

Bowler I.M. (1993) Stereotypes of women of Asian descent in midwifery: some evidence. *Midwifery*, **9**(1): 7–16.

British Pain Society (2005a) *Recommendations for the appropriate use of opioids in persistent non-cancer pain*, http://www.britishpainsociety.org/book_opioid_main.pdf.

British Pain Society (2005b) *Spinal cord stimulation for the management of pain*, http://www.britishpainsociety.org/book_scs_main.pdf.

British Pain Society (2007) *Intrathecal drug delivery for the management of pain and spasticity in adults: recommendations for best clinical practice*, http://www.britishpainsociety.org/book_ittd_main.pdf.

Brockopp D., Brockopp G., Warden S., Wilson J., Carpenter J. et al. (1998) Barrier to change: a pain management project. *International Journal of Nursing Studies*, **35**: 226–32.

Brody H. and Brody D. (2001) *The Placebo Response: How You Can Release the Body's Inner Pharmacy for Better Health*. London, Harper Perennial.

Bruster S., Jarman B., Bosanquet N., Weston D., Erens R. et al. (1994) National survey of hospital patients. *British Medical Journal*, **309**: 1542–6.

Buchholz M., Karl H., Pomietto M. and Lynn A. (1998) Pain scores in infants: a modified infant pain scale versus visual analogue. *Journal of Pain and Symptom Management*, **15**: 117–24.

Bucknall T., Manias E. and Botti M. (2001) Acute pain management: implications of the scientific evidence for nursing practice in the postoperative context. *International Journal of Nursing Practice*, **7**: 266–73.

Buttner W. and Finke W. (2002) Analysis of behavioural and physiological parameters for the assessment of postoperative analgesic demand in newborns, infants and young children: a comprehensive report on seven consecutive studies. *Pediatric Anesthesia*, **10**(3): 303–18.

CAIPE (Centre for Advancement of Interprofessional Education) (1997) Interprofessional education: What, how and when? *CAIPE Bulletin* No 13, London.

Carbajal R., Puape A., Hoenn E., Lenclen R. and Olivier-Martin M. (1997) APN: evaluation behavioural scale of acute pain in newborn infants. *Archives of Pediatrics & Adolescent Medicine*, 4: 623–8.

Callesen T., Bech K. and Kehlet H. (1999) Prospective study of chronic pain after groin hernia repair. *British Journal of Surgery*, 86(12): 1528–31.

Carlson A. (2007) Hot and cold: tried and true ice and heat modalities still prove effective for acute and chronic pain. *Rehabilitation Management*, 20(10): 32–3.

Carr D. and Goudas L. (1999) Acute pain. *Lancet*, 353: 2051–8.

Carr E.C.J. (1990) Postoperative pain: patients' expectations and experiences. *Journal of Advanced Nursing*, 15: 89–100.

Carr E.C.J. (1997) Evaluating the use of a pain assessment tool and care plan: a pilot study. *Journal of Advanced Nursing*, 26(6): 1073–9.

Carr E.C.J. (2002) Refusing analgesics: using continuous improvement to improve pain management on a surgical ward. *Journal of Clinical Nursing*, 11: 743–52.

Carr E.C.J. and Thomas V.J. (1997) Anticipating and experiencing postoperative pain: the patients' perspective. *Journal of Clinical Nursing*, 6(3): 191–201.

Carr E.C.J., Brockbank K. and Barrett K. (2003) Improving pain management through interprofessional education: evaluation of a pilot project. *Learning in Health and Social Care*, 2(1): 6–17.

Carroll D. and Seers K. (1998) Relaxation for the relief of chronic pain: a systematic review. *Journal of Advanced Nursing*, 27(3): 476–87.

Carroll D., Moore R., McQuay H., Fairman F., Tramer M. et al. (2000) Transcutaneous electrical nerve stimulation (TENS) for chronic pain. *Cochrane Database of Systemic Reviews*, http://www.cochrane.org/reviews/en/ab003222.html.

Cassell E. (2004) *The Nature of Suffering and the Goals of Medicine*. Oxford, Oxford University Press.

Cavenagh J., Good P. and Ravenscroft P. (2006) Neuropathic pain: are we out of the woods yet? *Internal Medicine Journal*, 36: 251–5.

Cecilia B. (2000) Age and pain differences in pain management following coronary artery graft bypass surgery. *Journal of Gerontological Nursing*, 26: 7–13.

Cepeda M., Carr D., Lau J. and Alvarez H. (2004) Music for pain relief. *Cochrane Database of Systemic Reviews*, http://www.cochrane.org/reviews/en/ab004843.html.

Challapalli V., Tremont-Lukats I., McNicol E., Lau J. and Carr D. (2005) Systemic administration of local anaesthetic agents to relieve neuropathic pain. *Cochrane Database of Systemic Reviews*, Oct 19 (4) CD003345.

Charatan F. (2001) New law requires doctors to learn care of the dying. *British Medical Journal*, 323(7321): 1088.

Cherkin D., Sherman K., Deyo R. and Shekelle P. (2003) A review of the evidence for the effectiveness, safety and cost of acupuncture, massage therapy and spinal manipulation for back pain. *Annals of Internal Medicine*, 138: 898–906.

Christensen J. (1993) *Nursing Partnership: A Model for Nursing Practice*. Edinburgh, Churchill Livingstone.

Cignacco E., Mueller R., Hamers J. and Gessler P. (2004) Pain assessment in the neonate using the Bernese Pain Scale for Neonates. *Early Human Development*, 78: 125–31.

Cignacco E., Hamers J., Stoffel L., VanLingen R., Gessler P. et al. (2007) The efficacy of non-pharmacological interventions in the management of procedural pain in preterm and term neonates: a systematic literature review. *European Journal of Pain*, 11: 139–52

Clarke E.B., French B., Bilodeau M.L., Capasso V.C., Edwards A. et al. (1996) Pain management knowledge, attitudes and clinical practice: the impact of nurses' characteristics and education. *Journal of Pain and Symptom Management*, 11(1): 18–31.

Clements S. and Cummings S. (1991) Helplessness and powerlessness: caring for clients in pain. *Holistic Nursing Practice*, 6(1): 76–85.

Cohen-Mansfield J. and Lipson S. (2002) Pain in cognitiviely impaired nursing home residents: how well are physicians diagnosing it? *Journal of American Geriatrics Society*, 50: 1039–44.

Cole J. (2004) *Still Lives: Narratives of Spinal Cord Injury*. Cambridge, MA, Bradford Book/MIT Press.

Corley M. and Goren, S. (1998). The dark side of nursing: impact of stigmatizing responses on patients. *Scholarly Inquiry for Nursing Practice*, 12(2): 99–122.

Corran T.M. and Melita B. (1998) Pain in later life. In Carter B. (ed.) *Perspectives on Pain: Mapping the Territory*. London, Arnold, pp. 243–63.

Covington E. (2000) Psychogenic pain: what it means, why it does not exist, and how to diagnose it. *Pain Medicine*, 1: 287–94.

Cowan D., White A. and Griffiths P. (2004) Use of strong opioids in the community for chronic non-cancer pain: a case study. *British Journal of Community Nursing*, 9(2): 53–8.

Cowan D., Wilson-Barnett J, Griffiths P. and Allan L. (2003) A survey of chronic non cancer pain patients prescribed opioid analgesics. *Pain Medicine*, 4(4): 340–51.

Craig K., Whitfield M., Grunau R., Linton J. and Hadjistavropoulos H. (1993) Pain in the preterm neonate: behavioural and physiological indices. *Pain*, 52: 287–99.

Crombie I, Davies H. and Macrae W. (1998) Cut and thrust: antecedent surgery and trauma among patients attending a chronic pain clinic, *Pain*, 76(1/2): 167–71.

Cuignet O., Pirson J., Soudon O. and Zizi M. (2007) Effects of gabapentin on morphine consumption and pain in severely burned patients. *Burns*, 33(1): 81–6.

Dalton J., Carlson J., Blau W., Lindley C., Greer S. et al. (2001) Documentation of pain assessment and treatment: How are we doing? *Pain Management Nursing*, 2(2): 54–64.

Daousi C, MacFarlane I, Woodward A, Nurmikko T, Bundred P. et al. (2004) Chronic painful peripheral neuropathy in an urban community: a controlled comparison of people with and without diabetes. *Diabetic Medicine*, 21: 976–82.

Davidhizar R. and Giger J. (2004) A review of the literature on care of clients in pain who are culturally diverse. *International Nursing Reviews*, 51: 47–55.

Davis S. (2004) *The Use of Pethidine for Pain Management in the Emergency Department*. New South Wales Therapeutic Advisory Group, www.clininfo.health.nsw.gov.au/nswtag/publications/posstats/Pethidinefinal.pdf.

De D. (2005) Sickle cell anaemia 2: management approaches of painful episodes. *British Journal of Nursing*, 14(9): 844–9.

De Rond M., de Wit R., van Dam F., van Campen B., den Hartog Y. et al. (1999) Daily pain assessment: value for nurses and patients. *Journal of Advanced Nursing*, 29: 436–44.

Debillon T., Zupan V., Ravault N., Magny J. and Dehan M. (2001) Development and initial validation of the EDIN scale, a new tool for assessing prolonged pain in preterm infants. *Archives of Disabled Child Fetal & Neonatal Edition*, 85: F36–F41.

Debley J., Carter E., Gibson R., Rosenfeld M. and Redding G. (2005) The prevalence of ibuprofen-sensitive asthma in children: a randomized controlled bronchoprovocation challenge study. *Journal of Pediatrics*, 147: 233–8.

DH (Department of Health) (1998) *The New National Health Service*. London, HMSO.

DH (Department of Health) (2001) *Valuing People: A New Strategy for Learning Disability for the 21st Century*. London, TSO.

DH (Department of Health) (2005) *Creating a Patient-led NHS: Delivering the NHS Improvement Plan*, http://www.dh.gov.uk/en/Publicationsandstatistics/Publications/PublicationsPolicyAndGuidance/DH_4106506.

Diego M., Field T. and Hernandez-Reif M. (2005) Vagal activity, gastric motility and weight gain in massaged preterm neonates. *Journal of Pediatrics*, 147: 50–5.

Dihle A., Bjolseth G. and Helseth S. (2006) The gap between saying and doing in postoperative pain management. *Journal of Clinical Nursing*, 15(4): 469–79.

Dr Foster (2004) *Adult Chronic Pain Management Services*, http://www.drfoster.co.uk/library/reports/painManagement.pdf.

Drayer R., Henderson J. and Reidenberg M. (1999) Barriers to better pain control in hospitalised patients. *Journal of Pain and Symptom Management*, 17(6): 434–40.

Duhn L. and Medves J. (2004) A systematic integrative review of infant pain assessment tools. *Advances in Neonatal Care*, 4(3): 126–40.

DWP (Department of Work and Pensions) (2008) *No one Written off: Reforming Welfare to Reward Responsibility*, Green Paper, Cm 7363. London, TSO.

Eccleston C.C., de Williams C. and Stainton Rogers W. (1997) Patients' and professionals' understandings of the causes of chronic pain: blame, responsibility and identity protection. *Social Science & Medicine*, **45**(5): 699–709.

Eckhard K., Ammon S., Schanzle G., Mikus G. and Eichelbaum M. (1998) Same incidence of adverse drug events after codeine administration irrespective of the genetically determined differences in morphine formation. *Pain*, 76(1/2): 27–33.

Eide P. (2000) Wind-up and the NMDA receptor complex from a clinical perspective. *European Journal of Pain*, **4**(1): 5–15.

Elliott A., Smith B., Penny K., Smith W. and Chambers W. (1999) The epidemiology of chronic pain in the community. *Lancet*, **354**(9186): 1248–52.

Elliott T.E. and Elliott B.A. (1992) Physicians' attitudes and beliefs about use of morphine for cancer pain. *Journal of Pain and Symptom Management*, 7: 141–8.

eMedicine (2006) Muchausen syndrome, www.emedicine.com/emerg/topic830.htm.

Eriksen J., Jensen M., Sjøgren P., Ekholm O. and Rasmussen N. (2003) Epidemiology of chronic non-malignant pain in Denmark. *Pain*, **106**(3): 221–8.

Ernst E., De Smet P., Shaw D. and Murray V. (1998) Traditional remedies and the 'test of time'. *European Journal of Clinical Pharmacology*, **54**(2): 99–100.

Ernst E., Pittler M., Stevinson C. and White A. (2001) *The Desktop Guide to Complementary and Alternative Medicine*. Edinburgh, Mosby.

Esselman P., Thombs B., Magyar-Russell G. and Fauerbach J. (2006) Burn rehabilitation: state of the science. *American Journal of Physical Medicine Rehabilitation*, **85**: 383–414.

European Haemoglobinopathy Registry (2006) http://www.hbregistry.org.uk/.

Evans J.M., McMahon A., McGilchrist M. et al. (1995) Topical non-steroidal anti-inflammatory drugs and admission to hospital for upper gastrointestinal bleeding and perforation: a record lineage case-control study. *British Medical Journal*, **311**: 22–6.

Evans R. (1992) Some observations on whiplash injuries. *Clinical Neurology*, **10**(4): 975–97.

Fagerhaugh S. and Strauss A. (1977) *Politics of Pain Management: Staff-Patient Interaction*. London, Addison-Wesley.

Fallon M. (1997) Opioid rotation: does it have a role. *Palliative Medicine*, **11**: 177–8.

Feldt K. (2000) The checklist of nonverbal pain indicators (CNPI). *Pain Management Nursing*, **1**: 13–21.

Filitz J., Griessinger N., Sittl R., Likar R., Schüttler J. et al. (2005) Effects of intermittent hemodialysis on buprenorphine and norbuprenorphine plasma concentrations in chronic pain patients treated with transdermal buprenorphine. *European Journal of Pain*, **10**(8): 743–8.

Finnerup N. and Jensen T. (2004) Spinal cord injury pain: mechanisms and treatment. *European Journal of Neurology*, **11**: 73–82.

Fishbain D. (1994) Secondary gain concept: definition problems and its abuse in medical practice. *APS Journal*, **3**(4): 264–73.

Fitzgerald M. (1993) Development of pain pathways and mechanisms. In Anand K.J. and McGrath P.J. (eds) *Pain in Neonates*. Elsevier, Amsterdam, pp. 19–37.

Fitzpatrick R. (2004) It is time we shared good practice in supplementary prescribing. *Hospital Pharmacist*, **12**(5): 182–3.

Flaskerud J., Lesser J., Dixon E., Adnerson N., Conde F. et al. (1999) Health disparities among vulnerable populations: evolution of knowledge over five decades in nursing research publications. *Nursing Research*, **51**(2): 74–85.

Foley D. and McCutcheon H. (2004) Detecting pain in people with an intellectual disability. *Accident and Emergency Nursing*, **12**: 196–299.

Foley K.M. (1993) Pain assessment and cancer pain syndromes. In Doyle D., Hanks G.W. and MacDonald N. (eds) *Oxford Textbook of Palliative Medicine*. Oxford, Oxford Medical Publications, Chapter 4.

Forrest D. (1989) The experience of caring. *Journal of Advanced Nursing*, **14**: 815–23.

Forsyth D. (2007) Pain in patients with cognitive impairment. In Crome P., Main C. and Lally F. (eds) *Pain in Older People*. Oxford, Oxford University Press, Chapter 3.

Francke A.L. and Theeuwen I. (1994) Inhibition in expressing pain: a qualitative study among Dutch surgical breast cancer patients. *Cancer Nursing*, **17**(3): 193–9.

Friedman D.P. (1990) Perspectives on the medical use of drug abuse. *Journal of Pain and Symptom Management*, **5**: S2–S5.

Friedrichs J., Young S., Gallagher D., Keller C. and Kimura R. (1995) Where does it hurt? An interdisciplinary approach to improving the quality of pain assessment and management in the neonatal intensive care unit. *Nursing Clinics of North America*, **30**: 143–59.

Fries B., Simon S., Morris J., Flodstrom C. and Bookstein F. (2001) Pain in U.S. nursing homes: validating a pain scale for the minimum data set. *Gerontologist*, **41**: 173–9.

Fuchs-Lacelle S. and Hadjistavropoulos T. (2004) Development and preliminary validation of the pain assessment checklist for seniors with limited ability to communicate (PACSLAC). *Pain Management Nursing*, **5**: 37–49.

Funnell P. (1995) Exploring the value of interprofessional shared learning. In Soothill K., Mackay L. and Webb C. (eds) *Interprofessional Relations in Health Care*. London, Edward Arnold, pp. 163–71.

Gallego O., Baro G. and Arranz E. (2007) Oxycodone: a pharmacological and clinical review. *Clinical & Translational Oncology*, **9**(5): 298–307.

Gallo A. (2003) The fifth vital sign: implementation of the Neonatal Infant Pain Scale. *Journal of Obstetric, Gynecologic and Neonatal Nursing*, **32**(2): 199–206.

Ganier J., van Tulder M., Berman B. and Bambardier C. (2006) Herbal medicine for low back pain, *Cochrane Database of Systemic Reviews*, http://www.cochrane.org/reviews/en/ab004504.html.

Gatchel R. (2004) Psychosocial factors that can influence the self-assessment of function. *Journal of Occupational Rehabilitation*, **14**(3): 197–206.

Gatchel R. and Epkar J. (1999) Psychological predictors of chronic pain and response to treatment. In Gatchel R. and Turk D. (eds) *Psychosocial Factors in Pain*. New York, Guildford Press, pp. 412–34.

Gear R., Gordon N., Hossaini-Zadeh M., Lee J., Miaskowski C. et al. (2008) A subanalgesic dose of morphine eliminates nalbuphine anti-analgesia in postoperative pain. *Journal of Pain*, **9**(4): 337–41.

Gibson S. and Farrel M. (2004) A review of age differences in the neurophysiology of nociception and the perceptual experience of pain. *Clinical Journal of Pain*, **20**(4): 227–39.

Gibson S.J. and Helme R.D. (1995) Age difference in pain perception and report: a review of physiological, psychological, laboratory and clinical studies. In Budd K. and Hamann W. (eds) *Pain Reviews*, vol. 2. London, Edward Arnold, pp. 111–37.

Gilmartin J. (2007) Day surgery: patients' perceptions of a nurse-led preadmission clinic. *Journal of Clinical Nursing*, **13**(2): 243–50.

Gilmartin J. and, Wright K. (2007) The nurse's role in day surgery: a literature review. *International Nursing Review*, **54**(2): 183–90.

Gilson A.M., Maurer M.A. and Joranson D. (2005) State policy affecting pain management: recent improvements and the positive impact of regulatory health policies, *Health Policy*, http://www.medsch.wisc.edu/painpolicy/publicat/05hlthpol/05hlthpol.pdf.

Glajchen M. and Bookbinder M. (2001) Knowledge and perceived competence of home care nurses in pain management: a national survey. *Journal of Pain and Symptom Management*, **21**(4): 307–16.

Golianu B., Krane E., Seybold J., Almgren C. and Anand K. (2007) Non-pharmacological techniques for pain management in neonates. *Seminars in Perinatology*, **31**: 318–22.

Gordon D., Pellino T., Miaskowski C., McNeill J., Paice J. et al. (2002) A 10-year review of quality improvement monitoring in pain management: recommendations for standardized outcome measures. *Pain Management Nursing*, **3**: 116–30.

Gosline A. (2004) Hypnosis really changes your mind. *New Scientist*, **13**: 28, http://www.newscientist.com/article/dn6385-hypnosis-really-changes-your-mind.html.

Green C., Anderson K., Baker T. and Campbell S. (2003) The unequal burden of pain: confronting racial and ethnic disparities in pain. *Pain Medicine*, **4**(3): 277–94.

Greipp M.E. (1992) Undermedication for pain: an ethical model. *Advances in Nursing Science*, **15**(1): 44–53.

Grunau R., Oberlander T., Holsti L. and Whitfield, M. (1998) Bedside application of the Neonatal Facial Coding System in pain assessment of premature infants. *Pain*, **76**(3): 277–86.

Guay J. (2006) The benefits of adding epidural analgesia to general anaesthesia: a meta analysis. *Journal of Anaesthesia*, **20**(4): 335–40.

Gudin J. (2004) Expanding our understanding of central sensitization. *Medscape Neurology and Neurosurgery*, http://www.medscape.com/viewarticle/481798.

Guinsburg R., Kopelman B., Anand K., de Almeida M. and de Araujo Peres C. (1998) Physiological, hormonal and behavioural responses to a single fentanyl dose in intubated and ventilated preterm neonates. *Journal of Pediatrics*, **132**: 954–9.

Gunningberg L. and Idvall E. (2007) The quality of postoperative pain management from the perspective of patients, nurses and patients records. *Journal of Nursing Management*, **15**: 756–66.

Gustorff B., Dorner T., Likar R., Grisold W., Lawrence K. et al. (2008) Prevalence of self-reported neuropathic pain and impact on quality of life: a prospective representative survey. *Acta Anaesthesiologica Scandinavica*, **52**(1): 132–6.

Gymrek R. and Dahdah M. (2007) Regional anaesthesia and regional nerve block anaesthesia, http://www.emedicine.com/derm/TOPIC824.HTM.

Hadjistavropoulus H. and Shymkiw J. (2007) Predicting readiness to self-manage pain. *Clinical Journal of Pain*, **23**(3): 259–66.

Hall P. (2005) *A New Pain Manifesto: Pain, the 5th Vital Sign*. Chronic Pain Policy Coalition, http://www.paincoalition.org.uk/pain5.html.

Hammonds W., Brena S. and Unikel I. (1978) Compensation for work-related injuries and rehabilitation of patients with chronic pain. *Southern Medical Journal*, **71**(6): 664–5.

Harper P., Ersser S. and Gobbi M. (2007) How military nurses rationalize their postoperative pain assessment decisions. *Journal of Advanced Nursing*, **56**(6): 601–11.

Hawkins R. and Hart A. (2003) The use of thermal biofeedback in the treatment of pain associated with endometriosis: preliminary findings. *Applied Psychophysiology and Biofeedback*, **28**(4): 279–89.

Herr K., Bjoro K. and Decker S. (2006) Tools for assessment of pain in nonverbal older adults with dementia: a state-of-the-science review. *Journal of Pain and Symptom Management*, **31**(2): 170–92.

Hester J. (2007) The forgotten majority: pain in the older person. British Geriatric Society newsletter, http://www.bgsnet.org.uk/jan07nl/18-pain.htm.

Higgins J., Madjar I. and Walton J. (2004) Chronic pain in elderly nursing home residents: the need for nursing leadership. *Journal of Nursing Management*, **12**: 167–73.

Hodgkinson K., Bear M., Thorn J. and Van Blaricum S. (1994) Measuring pain in neonates: evaluating an instrument and developing a common language, *Australian Journal of Advanced Nursing*, **12**: 17–22.

Hoffman H., Patterson D., Carrougher G. and Sharar S. (2001) Effectiveness of virtual reality-based pain control with multiple treatments. *Clinical Journal of Pain*, **17**(3): 229–35.

Hollingshead J., Duhmke R. and Cornblath D. (2006) Tramadol for neuropathic pain. *Cochrane Database of Systematic Reviews*, Jul. http://mrw.interscience.wiley.com/cochrane/clsysrev/articles/CD003726/frame.html.

Horgan M. and Choonara I. (1996) Measuring pain in neonates: an objective score. *Pediatric Nursing*, **8**: 24–7.

Howarth A. (2005) Benefits of aromatherapy in the management of chronic pain. *Nursing Standard*, **19**(17): 20–1.

Hudcova J., McNicol E., Quah C., Lau J. and Carr D. (2006) Patient controlled opioid analgesia versus conventional opioid analgesia for postoperative pain. *Cochrane Database of Systematic Review*, http://www.cochrane.org/reviews/en/ab003348.html.

Hudson-Barr D., Capper-Michel B., Lambert S., Palermo T., Morbeto K. et al. (2002) Validation of the Pain Assessment in Neonates (PAIN) with the scale the Neonatal Infants Pain Scale (NIPS). *Neonatal Network*, **21**(6): 15–21.

Hurley A., Volicer B., Hanrahan P., Houde S. and Volicer L. (1992) Assessment of discomfort in advanced Alzheimer patients. *Research in Nursing & Health*, **15**: 369–77.

Hutchcroft B. and Peakcock J. (1999) The patient's perception of chronic pain. *Professional Nurse*, **15**(1): 26–30.

Im E., Guevara E. and Chee W. (2007) The pain experience of Hispanic patients with cancer in the United States. *Oncology Nursing Forum*, **34**(4): 861–8.

Institute for Cancer Research and the Royal Marsden Hospital (2008) 'Breaking Barriers: Management of Cancer-related Pain', CD-ROM. For further information, contact the Interactive Education Unit at the Institute of Cancer Research at ieu@icr.ac.uk or visit http://ieu.icr.ac.uk.

International Association for the Study of Pain (1986) Classification of chronic pain. Descriptions of chronic pain syndromes and definitions of pain terms. *Pain* (Supplement 3): S1–S226.

International Association for the Study of Pain/European Federation of IASP (2004) *Chapters. Fact Sheet: Unrelieved Pain is a Major Global Healthcare Problem*, http://www.painreliefhumanright. com/pdf/04a_global_day_fact_sheet.pdf.

Irajpour A., Norman I. and Griffiths P. (2006) Interprofessional education to improve pain management. *British Journal of Community Nursing*, 11(1): 29–32.

Ives M. (2007) Model empathy and respect when immunizing children who fear needles. *Canadian Nurse*, April: 6–7

Izard C. (1995) *The Maximally Discriminative Facial Movement Coding System*, 3rd edn. Neward, DE, University of Delaware.

Jacox A., Ferrell B. and Heidrich G. (1992) Managing acute pain: a guideline for the nation. *American Journal of Nursing*, 92(5): 49–55.

Jacox A., Carr D.B., Payne R. et al. (1994) *Management of Cancer Pain*. Clinical Practice Guideline No. 9, AHCPR Pub. No. 94–0592. Rockville, MD, Agency for Health Care Policy and Research, Public Health Service, US Department of Health and Human Services.

Jage J. (2005) Opioid tolerance and dependence: do they matter? *European Journal of Pain*, 9(2): 157–62.

Jankovic D. (ed.) (2004) *Regional Nerve Blocks and Infiltration Therapy*, 3rd edn. Oxford, Blackwell Publishing.

JCAHO (Joint Commission on Accreditation of Healthcare Organisations) (2000) *Standards for Pain and its Management*. Oakbrook Terrace, IL, JCAHO.

Jensen M. and Patterson D. (2006) Hypnotic treatment of chronic pain. *Journal of Behavioural Medicine*, 29(1): 95–124.

Johnson L. (2004) Managing acute and chronic pain in sickle cell disease. *Nursing Times*, 8(101): 40–3.

Joranson D. and Ryan K. (2007) Ensuring opioid availability: methods and resources. *Journal of Pain Symptom Management*, 33(5): 527–32.

Joyce B., Schade J., Keck J., Gerkensmeyer J., Raftery T. et al. (1994) Reliability and validity of preverbal pain assessment tools. *Issues of Comprehensive Pediatric Nursing*, 17(3): 121–35.

Kaki A., El-Yaski A. and Youseif E. (2005) Identifying neuropathic pain among patients with chronic low-back pain: use of the Leeds Assessment of Neuropathic Symptoms and Signs pain scale. *Regional Anesthesia and Pain Medicine*, 30(5): 422–9.

Karoly P., Ruehlman L., Aiken L., Todd M. and Newton C. (2006) Evaluating chronic pain impact among patients in primary care: further validation of a brief assessment instrument. *Pain Medicine*, 7(4): 289–98.

Kaye K., Welch S., Graudins L. and Graudins A. (2005) Pethidine in emergency departments: promoting evidence-based prescribing. *PharmacoEconomics and Outcomes News*, 183: 129–33, http://www. mja.com.au/public/issues/183_03_010805/kay10502_fm.pdf.

Kehlet H. (1997) Multimodal approach to control postoperative pathophysiology and rehabilitation. *British Journal of Anaesthesia*, 78: 606–17.

Kehlet H. and Dahl J. (2003) Anaesthesia, surgery and challenges in postoperative recovery. *Lancet*, 362(9399): 1921–8.

Kehlet H. and Holte K. (2001) Effect of postoperative analgesia on surgical outcome. *British Journal of Anaesthesia*, 87(1): 62–72

Kehlet H., Jensen T. and Woolf C. (2006) Persistent postsurgical pain: risk factors and prevention. *Lancet*, 367: 1618–25.

Keogh E., McCracken L. and Eccleston C. (2005) Do men and women differ in their response to interdisciplinary chronic pain management? *Pain*, 114: 37–46.

Kerns R., Rosenberg R. and Jacob M. (1994) Anger expression and chronic pain. *Journal of Behavioural Medicine*, 17: 57–67.

Kerr D., Cunningham C. and Wilkinson H. (2006) *Responding to the Pain Experiences of People with a Learning Difficulty and Dementia*. York, Joseph Rowntree Foundation.

Knotkova H. and Pappagallo M. (2007) Adjuvant analgesics. *Medicine Clinics of North America*, 91(1): 113–24.

Kober S., Scheck T., Greher M., Lieba F., Fleischhackl R. et al. (2002) Prehospital analgesia with acupressure in victims of minor trauma: a prospective, randomized, double-blinded trial. *Anaesthesia & Analgesia*, 95(3): 723–7.

Koh P. and Thomas V.J. (1994) Patient-controlled analgesia (PCA): does time saved by PCA improve patient satisfaction with nursing care? *Journal of Advanced Nursing*, 20(1): 61–70.

Kong J., Kaptchuk T., Polich G., Kirsch I. and Gollub R. (2007) Placebo analgesia: findings from brain imaging studies and emerging hypotheses. *Review of Neuroscience*, 18(3/4): 173–90.

Kong V. and Irwin M. (2007) Gabapentin: a multimodal perioperative drug? *British Journal of Anaesthesia*, 99(6): 775–86.

Kovach C., Weissman D., Griffie J., Matson S. and Muchka S. (1999) Assessment and treatment of discomfort for people with late-stage dementia. *Journal of Pain Symptom Management*, 18: 412–19.

Kracke G., Uthoff T. and Tobias S. (2005) Sugar solution analgesia: the effect of glucose on expressed Mu opioid receptors. *Anesthesia & Analgesia*, 101: 64–8.

Kradin R. (2008) *The Placebo Response and the Power of Unconscious Healing*. New York, Routledge Taylor & Francis.

Krechel S.W. and Bilner J. (1995) CRIES: a new neonatal postoperative pain measurement score. Initial testing of validity and reliability. *Paediatric Anaesthesia*, 5: 53–61.

Kurth T., Glynn R., Walker A., Chan K., Buring J. et al. (2003) Inhibition of clinical benefits of aspirin on first myocardial infarction by nonsteroidal anti-inflammatory drugs. *Circulation*, 108(10): 1191–5.

Laffey J., Coleman M. and Boylan J. (2000) Patients' knowledge of perioperative care. *Irish Journal of Medical Science*, 169(2): 113–18.

Lander J. (1990) Clinical judgements in pain management. *Pain*, 42: 15–22.

Lang T., Hager H., Funovits V., Barker R., Steinlechner B. et al. (2007) Prehospital analgesia with acupressure at the Baihui and Hegu points in patients with radial fractures: a prospective, randomized, double-blind trial. *American Journal of Emergency Medicine*, 25(8): 887–93.

Lasch K., Greenhill A., Wilkes G., Carr D., Lee M. et al. (2002) Why study pain? A qualitative analysis of medical and nursing faculty and students' knowledge of and attitudes to cancer pain management. *Journal of Palliative Medicine*, 5(1): 57–71.

Latham J. (1989) *Pain Control*. London, Austin Cornish.

Lawrence J., Alcock D., McGrath P., Kay J. and MacMurray S. (1993) The development of a tool to assess neonatal pain. *Neonatal Network*, 12: 59–66.

Layzell M. (2005) Improving the management of postoperative pain. *Nursing Times*, 101(26): 34–36.

Layzell M. (2007) Pain management: setting up a nurse-led femoral nerve block service. *British Journal of Nursing*, 16(2): 702–5.

Leape L., Berwick D. and Bates D. (2002) What practices will most improve safety? Evidence-based medicine meets patient safety. *Journal of the American Medical Association*, 288: 501–7.

Lefebvre-Chapiro S. and the Doloplus Group (2001) The Doloplus 2 scale: evaluating pain in the elderly. *European Journal of Palliative Care*, 8: 191–4.

Lewindon P.J., Harkness L. and Lewindon N. (1998) Randomised controlled trial of sucrose by mouth for the relief of infant crying after immunisation. *Archives of Disease in Childhood*, 78: 453–6.

Liebeskind J.C. and Melzack R. (1987) The international pain foundation: meeting a need for education in pain management. *Pain*, 30: 1–2.

Linton S.J. (1994) Chronic back pain: integrating psychological and physical therapy: an overview. *Behavioural Medicine*, 20: 101–4.

Loeb J. (1999) Pain management in long-term care. *American Journal of Nursing*, 99(2): 48–52.

McCaffrey B. and Ferrell B (1997) Nurses' knowledge of pain assessment and management: how much progress have we made? *Journal of Pain and Symptom Management*, 14(3): 175–88.

McCaffery M. and Beebe A. (1989) *Pain: Clinical Manual for Nursing Practice*. St Louis, CV Mosby.

McCaffery M. and Beebe A. (1994) *Pain: A Clinical Manual for Nursing Practice*, 2nd edn. London, CV Mosby.

McCaffery M. and Robinson E. (2002) Your patient is in pain: here's how you respond. *Nursing*, 32(10): 36–45.

McCaffrey R. and Freeman E. (2003) Effect of music on chronic osteoarthritis pain in older people. *Journal of Advanced Nursing*, 44(5): 517–24.

McGrath P. (1989) Evaluating a child's pain. *Journal of Pain and Symptom Management*, **4**(4): 198–214.

McGrath P.J., Johnson G., Goodman J.T., Schillinger J., Dunn J. et al. (1985) CHEOPS: a behavioural scale for rating postoperative pain in children. In Fields H.L., Dubner R. and Cervero F. (eds) *Advances in Pain Research and Therapy*. New York, Raven Press, pp. 395–402.

McHugh G. and Thoms G. (2002) The management of pain following day-case surgery. *Anaesthesia*, **57**(3): 270–5.

Mackintosh C. (2007) Assessment and management of patients with post-operative pain. *Nursing Standard*, **22**(5): 49–55.

McLean S., Clauw D., Abelson J. and Liberzon I. (2005) The development of persistent pain and psychological morbidity after motor vehicle collision: integrating the potential role of stress response systems into a biopsychosocial model. *Psychosomatic Medicine*, **67**(5): 783–90.

McMahon S. and Kolzenburg M. (eds) (2005) *Wall and Melzack's Textbook of Pain*, 5th edn. Edinburgh, Churchill Livingstone.

McQuay H. (2004) Antidepressants in chronic pain, http://www.jr2.ox.ac.uk/bandolier/booth/painpag/wisdom/adbmj2.html.

McQuay H. and Moore A. (1998) *An Evidence-based Resource for Pain Relief*. Oxford, Oxford University Press.

McQuay H., Moore A. and Justins D. (1997) Clinical review: treating pain in hospital. *British Medical Journal*, **314**: 1531–5.

McQuay H.J., Moore R.A., Eccleston C., Morley S. and Williams A.C. (1997) Systematic review of outpatient services for chronic pain control. *Health Technology Assessment*, **1**(6): 1–236.

Madjar I. (1998) *Giving Comfort and Inflicting Pain*. Edmonton, Alberta, Qual Institute Press.

Maguire P. and Pitceathly C. (2002) Key communication skills and how to acquire them. *British Medical Journal*, **325**: 697–700.

Manchikanti L., Fellows B., Pampati V., Damron C. and Barnhill R. (2002) Comparison of psychological status of chronic pain patients and the general population. *Pain Physician*, **5**(1): 40–8.

Mann E. (2003) Chronic pain and opioids; dispelling myths and exploring the facts. *Professional Nurse*, **18**(7): 408–11.

Mann E. and Carr E. (2006) *Pain Management*. Oxford, Blackwell Science.

Mann E. and Redwood S. (2000) Improving pain management: breaking down the invisible barrier. *British Journal of Nursing*, **9**(19): 2067–72.

Marcer D. and Deighton S. (1988) Intractable pain: a neglected area of medical education in the U.K. *Journal of the Royal Society of Medicine*, **81**: 698–700.

Marzinski L. (1991) The tragedy of dementia: clinically assessing pain in the confused, non-violent elderly. *Journal of Gerontological Nursing*, **6**(6): 25–8.

Medicines and Healthcare Products Regulatory Agency (2007), http://www.mhra.gov.uk/home/idcplg?IdcService=SS_GET_PAGE&nodeId=5.

Meinhart N.T. and McCaffery M. (1983) *Pain: A Nursing Approach to Assessment and Analysis*. Norwalk, CO, Appleton Century Crofts.

Melzack R. (1987) The short-form McGill Pain Questionnaire. *Pain*, **30**: 191–7.

Melzack R. (1999) From the gate to the neuromatrix. *Pain*, Aug, Suppl 6: S121–6.

Melzack R. and Katz J. (1994) Pain measurement in persons in pain. In Wall P.D. and Melzack R. (eds) *Textbook of Pain*, 3rd edn. Edinburgh, Churchill Livingstone, pp. 337–56.

Melzack R. and Torgerson W. (1971) On the language of pain. *Anaesthesiology*, **34**(1): 50–9.

Melzack R. and Wall P. (1965) Pain mechanisms: a new theory. *Science*, **150**: 971–9.

Melzack R. and Wall P. (1996) *The Challenge of Pain*, 2nd edn. Harmondsworth, Penguin.

Merkel S., Voepel-Lewis T., Shayevitz J. and Malviya S. (1997) Practice applications of research. The FLACC: a behavioural scale for scoring postoperative pain in young children. *Pediatric Nursing*, **23**: 293–97.

Merskey H. and Bogduk N. (1994) *Classification of Chronic Pain: Description of Chronic Pain Syndromes and Definitions of Pain Terms*, 2nd edn. Seattle, IASP Press.

Mico J., Ardid D., Berrocoso E. and Eschalier A. (2006) Antidepressants and pain. *Trends in Pharmacological Science*, **27**(7): 348–54.

Middleton C. (2004) Barriers to the provision of effective pain management. *Nursing Times*, **100**(3): 42–5.

Molton I., Graham C., Stoelb B. and Jensen M. (2007) Current psychological approaches to the management of chronic pain. *Current Opinion in Anaesthesiology*, **20**(5): 485–9.

Mongin G. (2007) Tramadol extended-release formulations in the management of pain due to osteoarthritis. *Expert Review of Neurotherapeutics*, 7(12): 1775–84.

Moore A. and McQuay H. (2005) Acupuncture: not just needles? *Lancet*, **366**(9480): 100–1.

Moores Y. (1999) Clinical governance and nursing. *Professional Nurse*, **15**(2): 74–5.

Morgan M., and Horne R. (2005) Explaining patients' behaviour. In report for the National Co-ordinating Centre for NHS Service Delivery and Organisation R&D, *Concordance, Adherence and Compliance in Medicine Taking*. London, NCCSDO, pp. 39–60.

Morrison R. and Siu A. (2000) A comparison of pain and its treatment in advanced dementia and cognitively intact patients with hip fracture. *Journal of Pain & Symptom Management*, **19**: 240–8.

Murat I. (2003) Procedural pain in children: evidence-based best practice and guidelines. *Regional Anaesthesia and Pain Medicine*, **28**(6): 561–72.

Nagi H. (2004) Acute pain services in the United Kingdom. *Acute Pain*, **5**(3/4): 89–107.

Nagle C.J. and McQuay H. (1990) Opioid receptors; their role in effect and side-effect. *Current Anaesthesia and Critical Care*, **1**: 247–52.

Nagy S. (1998) A comparison of the effects of patients' pain on nurses working in burns and neonatal intensive care units. *Journal of Advanced Nursing*, **27**(2): 335–40.

National Prescribing Centre (2004) *Patient Group Directions: A Practical Guide and Framework of Competencies for all Professionals using Patient Group Directions*, http://www.npc.co.uk/publications/pgd/pgd.pdf.

NLH Learning Disabilities Specialist Library (2007) *Clinical question and answer: What assessments are available to assess pain in people with a learning disability?*, www.library.nhs.uk/learningdisabilities/viewResource.aspx?resID=259948.

NMC (Nursing and Midwifery Council) (2004) *Code of Professional Conduct*, http://www.nmc-uk.org/aFrameDisplay.aspx?DocumentID=201.

Notcutt W. (1997) Better to define and enhance the role of ward surgical nurses (letter). *British Medical Journal*, **314**: 1347.

O'Rorke, J. (2007) Physicians' comfort in caring for patients with chronic nonmalignant pain. *American Journal of the Medical Sciences*, **333**(2): 93–100.

Older C., Carr E. and Warr J. (2007) An exploration of patients decision-making following day case surgery. *Journal of Ambulatory Care*, **13**(1): 41–68, http://www.ambulatorysurgeryorg/.

Oyama O., Paltoo C. and Greengold J. (2007) Somatoform disorders. *American Family Physician*, **76**(9): 1333–8.

Page G. (2005) Surgery-induced immunosuppression and postoperative pain management. *AACN Clinical Issues*, **16**(3): 302–9.

Parmelee P.A. (1996) Pain in cognitively impaired older persons. In Ferrell B.A. (ed.) *Clinics in Geriatric Medicine: Pain Management*. Philadelphia, W.B. Saunders, pp. 473–87.

Payne R. (1989) Pain in the drug abuser. In Foley K and Payne R. (eds) *Current Therapy of Pain*. Philadelphia, BC Decker, pp. 46–54.

Pearson A. (ed.) (1988) *Primary Nursing*. London, Croom Helm.

Perkins F. and Kehlet H. (2000) Chronic pain as an outcome of surgery: a review of predictive factors. *Anaesthesiology*, **93**(4): 1123–33.

Peters J., Koot H., Grunau R., de Boer J., van Druenen M. et al. (2003) Neonatal facial coding system for assessing postoperative pain in infants: item reduction is valid and feasible. *Clinical Journal of Pain*, **19**(6): 353–63.

Picker Institute (2007) *A Hidden Problem: Pain in Older People*. Oxford, Picker Institute, http://www.pickereurope.org/Filestore/Publications/paincarehomes_final.pdf.

Pincus T., Vogel S., Burton A., Santos R. and Field A. (2006) Fear avoidance and prognosis in back pain: a systematic review and synthesis of current evidence. *Arthritis and Rheumatology*, **54**(12): 3999–4010.

Pokela M. (1994) Pain relief can reduce hypoxemia in distress neonates during routine treatment procedures. *Pediatrics*, 93: 379–83.

Porter J. and Jick H. (1980) Addiction rare in patients treated with narcotics. *New England Journal of Medicine*, 301: 419–26.

Potter J, Higginson I., Scadding J. and Quigley C. (2003) Identifying neuropathic pain in patients with head and neck cancer: use of the Leeds Assessment of Neuropathic Symptoms and Signs Scale. *Journal of the Royal Society of Medicine*, 96: 379–83.

Potter R.G. (1990) The frequency of presentation of pain in general practice: an analysis of 1000 consecutive consultations. *Journal of the Pain Society*, 8: 112–16.

Potter R.G. (1998) The prevention of chronic pain. In Carter B. (ed.) *Perspectives on Pain: Mapping the Territory*. London, Arnold, pp. 186–94.

Poyhia R and Kalso E. (1999) Pain related undergraduate teaching in medical faculties in Finland. *Pain*, 79(2/3): 121–5.

Raiman J. (1986) Pain relief: a two way process. *Nursing Times*, 82(15): 24–7.

Ranger M., Johnston C. and Anand K. (2007) Current controversies regarding pain assessment in neonates. *Seminar in Perinatology*, 31(5): 283–8.

RCN (Royal College of Nursing) (2000) *Clinical Practice Guidelines: the Recognition and Assessment of Acute Pain in Children: Technical Report*, http://www.rcn.org.uk/development/practice/clinicalguidelines/pain.

Ready L.B., Oden R., Chadwick H.S. et al. (1988) Development of an anaesthesiology-based postoperative pain management service. *Anaesthesiology*, 68: 100–6.

Regnard C., Reynolds J., Watson B., Matthews D., Gibson L. et al. (2007) Understanding distress in people with severe communication difficulties: developing and assessing the Disability Distress Assessment Tool (DisDAT). *Journal of Intellectual Disability Research*, 51(4): 277–92.

Reisner S.J. (1993) The era of the patient: using the experience of illness in shaping the missions of health care. *Journal of the American Medical Association*, 269(8): 1012–17.

Ren K., Anseloni V., Zou S., Wade E., Novikova S. et al. (2004) Characterization of basal and re-inflammation-associated long-term alteration in pain responsivity following short-lasting neonatal local inflamatory insult. *Pain*, 110(3): 588–96.

Richardson A. (1997) Cancer pain and its management. In Thomas V.N. (ed.) *Pain: Its Nature and Management*. London, Baillière Tindall, pp. 194–219.

Riley J., Eisenberg E., Muller-Schwefe G., Drewes A. and Arendt-Nielsen L. (2007) Oxycodone: a review of its use in the management of pain. *Current Medical Research and Opinion*, 24(1): 175–92, http://www.informapharmascience.com/.S.

Rohling M., Binder L. and Langhinrichsen-Rohling J. (1995) Money matters: a meta-analytic review of the association between financial compensation and the experience and treatment of chronic pain. *Health Psychology*, 14(6): 537–47.

Rolke R., Baron R., Maier C., Tolle T., Treede R. et al. (2006) Quantitative sensory testing in the German Research Network on Neuropathic Pain (DFNS): standardized protocol and reference values. *Pain*, 123(3): 231–43.

Rosenstein D. and Oster H. (1988) Differential facial responses for four basic tastes in newborns. *Child Development*, 59: 1555–68.

Royal College of Surgeons and College of Anaesthetists (1990) *Report of the Working Party on Pain after Surgery*. London, HMSO.

Ruda M., Qunig-Dong L., Hohmann A., Peng Y. and Tachibana T. (2000) Altered nociceptive neuronal circuits after neonatal peripheral inflammation. *Science*, 289: 628–30.

Sachs C. (2005) Oral analgesics for acute non-specific pain. *American Family Physician*, 71(5): 913–18.

Salerno E. (1995) Race, culture and medications. *Journal of Emergency Nurses*, 21: 560–2.

Sampson K. (2007) Is morphine a suitable analgesia for the ventilated neonate? A discussion of the research findings the alternatives and their implications upon neonatal intensive care. *Journal of Neonatal Nursing*, 13: 58–63.

Schade J., Joyce B., Gerkensmeyer J. and Keck J. (1996) Comparison of three preverbal scales for postoperative pain assessment in a diverse pediatric sample. *Journal of Pain Symptom Management*, **12**: 348–59.

Schafheutle E., Cantrill J. and Noyce P. (2001) Why is pain management suboptimal on surgical wards? *Journal of Advanced Nursing*, **33**(6): 728–37.

Schenk M., Putzier M., Kugler B., Tohtz S., Voigt K. et al. (2006) Postoperative analgesia after major spine surgery; patient-controlled epidural analgesia versus patient-controlled intravenous analgesia. *Anesthesia & Analgesia*, **103**(5): 1311–17.

Schoenwald A. and Clark G. (2006) Acute pain in surgical patients. *Contemporary Nurse*, **22**(1): 97–108.

Schofield P. (2002) Evaluating Snoezelen for relaxation with chronic pain management. *British Journal of Nursing*, **11**(12): 812–21.

Score M. and Attribute P. (2000) Physicians' attitudes toward pain and the use of opioid analgesics: results of a survey from the Texas Cancer Pain Initiative. *South Medical Journal*, **93**(5): 479–487, or Medscape.com.

Scott N.B. and Hodson M. (1997) Public perceptions of postoperative pain and its relief. *Anaesthesia*, **52**: 438–42.

Seers K. (1997) Chronic non-malignant pain: a community-based approach to management. In Thomas V.J. (ed.) *Pain: Its Nature and Management*. London, Baillière Tindall, pp. 220–37.

Seers K. and Friedli K. (1996) The patients' experiences of their chronic non-malignant pain. *Journal of Advanced Nursing*, **24**: 1160–8.

Shade P. (1992) PCA: can client education improve outcomes? *Journal of Advanced Nursing*, **17**: 408–13.

Sheridan R.L., Petras L., Lydon M. and Salvo P.M. (1997) Once-daily wound cleansing and dressing change: efficacy and cost. *Journal of Burn Care and Rehabilitation*, **18**(2): 139–40.

Sherwood G., Adams McNeill J., Starck P., Nieto B. and Thompson C. (2000) Qualitative assessment of hospitalised patients' satisfaction with pain management. *Research in Nursing and Health*, **23**: 486–95.

Sherwood G., Mcneill J., Hernandez L. and Penarrieta I. (2005) A multinational study of pain management among Hispanics: an evidence-based approach. *Journal of Research in Nursing*, **10**: 403–23.

Siddall P., Yezierski R. and Loeser J. (2000) Pain following spinal cord injury: clinical features, prevalence and taxonomy. *IASP Newsletter 3*, Seattle, IASP Press, http://www.iasp-pain.org/TC00-3.html.

Siddall P., Yezierski R. and Loeser J. (2002) Taxonomy and epidemiology of spinal cord injury pain. In Yezierski R. and Burchiel K. (eds) *Spinal Cord Injury Pain: Assessment, Mechanisms, Management*. Seattle, IASP Press, pp. 9–24.

Siedliecki S. and Good M. (2006) Effect of music on power, pain, depression and disability. *Journal of Advanced Nursing*, **54**(5): 553–62.

Sindhu F. (1996) Are non-pharmacological nursing interventions for the management of pain effective? A meta-analysis. *Journal of Advanced Nursing*, **24**(6): 1152–9.

Sjostrom B., Dahlgren L. and Haljame H. (2000) Strategies used in post-operative pain assessment and their clinical accuracy. *Journal of Clinical Nursing*, **9**: 111–18.

Skrabanek P. and McCormick J. (1990) *Follies and Fallacies in Medicine*. Buffalo, NY, Prometheus Books.

Sloman R., Rosen G., Rom M. and Shir Y. (2004) Nurses' assessment of pain in surgical patients: issues and innovations in nursing practice. *Journal of Advanced Nursing*, **52**(2): 125–32.

Sluka K.A. and Rees H. (1997) The neuronal response to pain. *Physiotherapy Theory and Practice*, **13**(1): 3–22.

Smeets R. and Wittink H. (2007) The deconditioning paradigm for chronic low back pain unmasked? *Pain*, **130**(3): 201–2.

Smith G. (1998) Audit and bridging the analgesic gap. *Anaesthesia*, **53**: 521–2.

Snow A., Weber J., O'Malley K., Cody M. and Beck C. (2004) NOPPAIN: a nursing assistant-administered pain assessment instrument for use in dementia. *Dementia & Geriatric Cognitive Disorders*, **17**: 240–6.

Soberman R. and Christmas P. (2003) The organization and consequences of eicosanoid signaling. *Journal of Clinical Investigation*, **111**: 1107–13.

Solomon L. (2008) Treatment and prevention of pain due to vaso-occlusive crises in adults with sickle cell disease: an educational void. *Blood*, **3**(3): 997–1003.

South M., Strauss R., South A., Boggess J. and Thorp J. (2005) The use of non-nutritive sucking to decrease the physiologic pain response during neonatal circumcision: a randomised controlled trial. *Obstetrics & Gynecology*, **193**: 537–43.

Sparshott M. (1996) The development of a clinical distress scale for ventilated newborn infants: identification of pain and distress based on validated behavioural scores. *Journal of Neonatal Nursing*, **2**: 5–11.

Spence K., Gillies D., Harrison D., Johnston L. and Nagy S. (2005) A reliable pain assessment tool for clinical assessment in the neonatal intensive care unit. *Journal of Obstetric, Gynecologic & Neonatal Nursing*, **34**(1): 80–86

Stallard P., Williams L., Lenton S. and Velleman R. (2001) Pain in cognitively impaired, non-communicating children. *Archives of Diseases in Childhood*, **85**(6): 460–2.

Stempien L. and Tsai T. (2000) Intrathecal baclofen pump use for spasticity: a clinical survey. *American Journal of Physical Medicine & Rehabilitation*, **79**(6): 536–41.

Stevens B., Yanada H. and Ohlsson A. (2004) Sucrose for analgesia in newborn infants undergoing painful procedures. *Cochrane Database of Systematic Reviews*, http://www.cochrane.org/reviews/en/ab001069.html.

Stevens B., Johnston C., Petryshen P. and Taddio A. (1996) Premature infant pain profile: development and initial validation. *Clinical Journal of Pain*, **12**(1): 13–22.

Stone A., Shiffman S., Schwartz J., Broderick J. and Hufford M. (2002) Patient non-compliance with paper diaries. *British Medical Journal*, **324**(7347): 1193–4.

Streetly A., Maxwell K. and Mejia A. (1997) *Sickle Cell Disorders in London: A Needs Assessment of Screening and Cure Services*. London, United Medical and Dental Schools Department of Public Health Medicine (Fair Shares for London report).

Streitberger K., Ezzo J. and Schneider A. (2006) Acupuncture for nausea and vomiting an update of clinical and experimental studies. *Autonomic Neuroscience*, **129**(1/2): 107–17.

Summer G., Puntillo K., Maiskowski C., Green P. and Levene J. (2007) Burn injury pain: the continuing challenge. *Journal of Pain*, **8**(7): 533–48.

Sutherland S. (1996) Procedural burn pain intensity under conditions of varying physical control by the patient. *Journal of Burn Care and Rehabilitation*, **17**(5): 457–63.

Svensson I., Sjöström B. and Haljamäe H. (2001) Influence of expectations and actual pain experiences on satisfaction with postoperative pain management. *European Journal of Pain*, **5**: 125–35.

Symonds, T.L., Burton, A.K., Tillotson, K.M. and Main, C.J. (1996) Do attitudes and beliefs influence work loss due to low back trouble? *Occupational Medicine*, **46**(1): 25–32.

Taddio A., Nulman I., Koren B., Stevens B. and Koren G. (1995) A revised measure of acute pain in infants. *Journal of Pain Symptom Management*, **10**: 456–63.

Taverner T. (2003) A regional pain management audit. *Nursing Times*, **99**(8): 34–7.

Taylor N.M., Hall G.M. and Salmon P. (1996) Patients' experiences of patient-controlled analgesia. *Anaesthesia*, **51**: 525–8.

Thomas V.J. and Rose F.D. (1993) Patient-controlled analgesia: a new method for old. *Journal of Advanced Nursing*, **18**: 1719–26.

Todd K., Green C., Bonham V., Haywood C. and Ivy E. (2006) Sickle cell disease related pain: crisis and conflict. *Journal of Pain*, **7**(7): 453–8.

Tölle T., Xu X. and Sadosky A. (2006) Painful diabetic neuropathy: a cross-sectional survey of health state impairment and treatment patterns. *Journal of Diabetes and its Complications*, **20**(1): 26–33.

Townsend A., Hunt K. and Wyke S. (2003) Managing multiple morbidity in mid-life: a qualitative study of attitudes to drug use. *British Medical Journal*, **327**(837): 348–9.

Tsao J. (2007) Effectiveness of massage therapy for chronic, non-malignant pain: a review. *Evidence-based Complementary. and Alternative. Medicine*, **4**(2): 165–79, http://ecam.oxfordjournals.org/cgi/content/full/4/2/165.

Turan A., Karamanlioglu B., Memis D., Hamamcioglu M., Tukenmez B. et al. (2004) Analgesic effects of gabapentin after spinal surgery. *Anesthesiology*, **100**(4): 935–8.

Turk D. and Okifuji A. (1996) Perception of traumatic onset, compensation status, and physical findings: impact on pain severity, emotional distress, and disability in chronic pain patients. *Journal of Behavioural Medicine*, **19**(5): 435–53.

Tyrer S.P. (1992) *Psychology, Psychiatry and Chronic Pain*. Oxford, Butterworth-Heinemann.

Tywcross R. (1999) Opioids. In Wall P. and Melzack R. (eds) *Textbook of Pain*, 4th edn. Edinburgh, Churchill Livingstone, pp. 1187–1214.

US Bureau of the Census (2004) *2004 American Community Survey*, http://factfinder.censua.gov/.

US Food and Drug Administration (2007) www.fda.gov/default.htm.

Valdix S. and Puntillo K. (1995) Pain, pain relief and accuracy of their recall after cardiac surgery. *Progress in Cardiovascular Nursing*, **10**: 3–11.

Vallerand A. and Polomano R. (2000) The relationship of gender to pain. *Pain Management Nursing*, **1**(3 Suppl 1): 8–15.

van den Beuken-van Everdingena M., de Rijkea J., Kesselsb A., Schoutenc H., van Kleefeld M. et al. (2007) High prevalence of pain in patients with cancer in a large population-based study in The Netherlands. *Pain*, **132**(3): 312–20.

van Dijk M, Peters JW, van Deventer P. and Tibboel D. (2005) The Comfort Behaviour Scale: a tool for assessing pain and sedation in infants. *American Journal of Nursing*, **105**(1): 33–6.

Van Twillert B., Bremer M. and Faber A. (2007) Computer-generated virtual reality to control pain and anxiety in pediatric and adult burn patients during wound dressing changes. *Journal of Burn Care & Research*, **28**(5): 694–702.

Villanueva M., Smith T., Erickson J., Lee A. and Singer C. (2003) Pain assessment for the dementing elderly (PADE): reliability and validity of a new measure. *Journal of American Medical Directors Association*, Jan/Feb 1–8.

Waddell G. (1992) Biopsychosocial analysis of low back pain. *Baillière's Clinical Rheumatology*, **6**: 523–51.

Waddell, G. (1997) Low back pain: a twentieth century health care enigma. In Jensen T.S., Turner A. and Weisenfeld-Hallin Z. (eds) *Progress in Pain Research and Management*, vol. 8. Seattle, International Association for the Study of Pain, pp. 101–12.

Wagner Anke A.G., Stenehjem A.E. and Stanghelle J.K. (1995) Pain and life quality within two years of spinal cord injury. *Paraplegia*, **33**: 555–9.

Wall P. (1992) The placebo effect: an unpopular topic. *Pain*, **51**: 1–3.

Wall P. (1999) *Pain: The Science of Suffering*. London, Weidenfeld & Nicolson.

Wall P. and Jones M. (1991) *Defeating Pain: The War against a Silent Epidemic*. New York, Plenum Press.

Wall P. and Melzack R. (1994) *Textbook of Pain*, 3rd edn, Edinburgh, Churchill Livingstone.

Wall P. and Melzack R. (1999) *Textbook of Pain*, 4th edn, Edinburgh, Churchill Livingstone.

Walsh D. (1997) *TENS: Clinical Applications and Related Theory*. Edinburgh, Churchill Livingstone.

Walsh D. and Radcliffe J. (2002) Pain beliefs and perceived physical disability of patients with chronic low back pain. *Pain*, **97**(1/2): 23–31.

Walsh, M. (1993) Pain and anxiety in A&E attenders. *Nursing Standard*, **7**: 40–2.

Warden V., Hurley A. and Volicer L. (2003) Development and psychometric evaluation of the pain assessment in advanced dementia (PAINAD) scale. *Journal of American Medical Directors Association*, Jan/Feb 9–15.

Watt-Watson J., McGillion M. and Hunter J. (2007) A survey of pain education in pre-licensure health science faculties in Canadian Universities. Canadian Pain Society, www.canadianpainsociety.ca/SurveyOfPainCurricula.pdf .

Watt-Watson J., Hunter J., Pennefather P., Librach L., Raman-Wilms L. et al. (2004) An integrated undergraduate pain curriculum, based on IASP curricula, for six health science faculties. *Pain*, **110**(1/2): 140–8.

Weber T., Matzl J., Rokintansky A., Klimscha W., Neumann K. et al. (2007) Superior postoperative pain relief with thoracic epidural analgesia versus intravenous patient-controlled analgesia after minimally invasive pectus excavatum repair. *Journal of Thoracic Cardiovascular Surgery*, **134**(4): 865–70.

Weiner D. and Rudy T. (2002) Attitudinal barriers to effective treatment of persistent pain in nursing home residents. *Journal of American Geriatrics Society*, **50**: 2035–40.

Weiner D., Peterson B. and Keefe F. (1998) Evaluating persistent pain in long term care residents: what role for pain maps? *Pain*, **76**: 249–57.

Weisenberg M. (1998) Cognitive aspects of pain and pain control. *International Journal of Clinical and Experimental Hypnosis*, **46**: 44–61.

WHO (World Health Organization) (1996) *Cancer Pain Relief*, 2nd edn. Geneva, WHO.

Widerstrom-Noga E., Felipe-Cuervo E. and Yezierski R. (2001) Chronic pain after spinal injury: interference with sleep and daily activities. *Archives of Physical Medicine & Rehabilitation*, **82**: 1571–7.

Wiesenfeld-Hallin Z. (2005) Sex differences in pain perception. *Gender Medicine*, **2**(3): 137–45.

Williamson A. and Hoggart B. (2005) Pain: a review of three commonly used pain rating scales. *Clinical Nursing*, **14**(7): 798–804.

Williamson-Smith A. (2007) Education and training of pain nurse specialists in the United Kingdom. *Acute Pain*, **9**(4): 207–13.

Wilson B. (2007) Nurses knowledge of pain. *Journal of Clinical Nursing*, **16**(6): 1012–20.

Windsor A.L., Glynn C.J. and Mason D.G. (1996) National provision of pain services. *Anaesthesia*, **51**: 228–31.

Wu C., Berenholtz S., Pronovost P. and Fleisher L. (2002) Systematic review and analysis of postdischarge symptoms after outpatient surgery. *Anesthesiology*, **96**(4): 994–1003.

Zborowski M. (1952) Cultural components and responses to pain. *Journal of Social Issues*, **8**(4): 16–30.

Zuccaroli J. and Van Schoor J. (2007) Abdominal pain. *Professional Nursing Today*, **11**(4): 35–8.

Index

A

A beta fibres 9–12, 20, 104, 107, 126, 127
A delta fibres 6–7, 89
accountability 68–9
acupressure 127, 163
acupuncture 127, 163
acute pain 4, 6–16
acute pain services 80–5
addiction 16, 93, 95–6, 180, 188, 189
    fear of 66
    pseudo-addiction 192
adjuvants 120–1
admission procedures 92
A&E departments 97
affective-motivational dimension 18–19, 22
age 117
agonist 16–17
algorithm 70
allodynia 20, 178
alternative therapy 126
amitriptyline 178
anaesthetist 65, 81
analgesics
    acute pain 86–95
    maximising prescription 98–9
    mild-to-moderate pain 86–9
anger 195
antagonist 16–17
anticonvulsants 122, 178
antidepressants 121, 178
antiemetic 99
antihypertensives 122
antispasmodic agents 122
anxiety 20, 104, 131, 176, 179, 181, 184
appendicitis 8
aromatherapy 130
around-the-clock dosing 99

arthritis 122, 125, 128, 129, 133, 134
aspirin 88
assessment
    advantages 28–9
    age 33–4
    community 30
    culture 32
    gender 34
    how to assess pain 29–32
    learning disabilities 155–6
    multidimensional tools 37–43
    neonates and preverbal children 34, 157–60
    neuropathic pain 38
    nurse factors 27, 32
    older people 146, 147, 150–4
    patient factors 32–3
    simple descriptive scales 35–6
    tools 35–49
    when to assess pain 29
asthma 88
atelectasis 79
autonomic 22, 104, 131

B

baclofen 122
balanced analgesia (see multimodal)
barriers to effective pain management
    healthcare professionals 56–9
    knowledge deficit 56–60
    lack of accountability 68–9
    organisational aspects 67
    patient factors 63–7
benzodiazepines 123
biliary colic 93
biofeedback 131
bisphosphonates 124
blackcurrent seeds 133
body language 30, 149–50
borage 133

bradykinin 13–14
brain-injured patients 155–6
Brief Pain Inventory 38–40
British Pain Society 96, 124, 129, 192
buprenorphine 16, 94
burns 173–7
buscopan 122

C

c fibres 8–9, 20, 104
cancer pain 4, 89, 122
capsaicin 123, 133
carbamazepine 122
ceiling effect 87
central inhibition 20
central pain 178
changing dressings 160, 174–5
changing practice 50–1, 70
charts for regular everyday use 43–5
chemotherapy 123
CHEOPS assessment tool 158
chest infection 30
childbirth 34, 166
chilli peppers 133 (*see also* capsaicin)
chronic pain 4, 113
    after surgery 77
    malignant 113
    non-malignant 113
    clinics 137–8
clinical governance 69
clinical nurse specialist 81
clinical psychologist 81
clonidine 122
codeine 89–90
cognitive aspects 11–12
cognitive-behavioural therapy 130
cognitive-evaluative dimension 18–19,
    22
cognitive impairment 149–54
cold therapy 129–30, 163
comfort 85, 105, 163
communication 45, 59, 148, 149
    verbal 29–30
compensation 192, 194
complementary approaches 126
confusion 92

controlled drugs 69–70
COX-2 88–9
CRIES assessment tool 160
culture 65–6
cyclo-oxygenase 13–14

D

deconditioning 80, 117, 184
deep vein thrombosis 30, 79, 85
definitions of pain 4–6, 113, 114
dementia 149
dependence 96
depression 136, 184, 186
Descartes' theory 2–3
devil's claw 133
diabetes 114, 125
diamorphine 92
diaries 43, 153
diazepam 123
dihydrocodeine 90
disability living allowance 193–4
disfigurement 174
distraction 12, 85, 105, 163
dorsal horn 6
dressing changes 106–7, 174–7
dynorphins 14–16
dysphoria 123

E

education 60–3, 65, 72, 81, 99, 180
    interprofessional 60
electronic patient record 182
EMLA cream 162
emotion 30
empathy 56, 135
endocrine 22
endogenous opioids 14–17
endometriosis 131
endorphins 14–16, 126, 128
enkephalins 14–16
entonox 97–8
epidural analgesia 81, 85, 101–3
    assessment 46–7
ethnic minorities 164–7 (*see also*
    culture)
evening primrose oil 133

evidence-based practice 67, 91
    strategies 166–7
exercise 135, 179

F

facial expression 30
    neonates 160
    older person 150
family 195
fast/first pain 6–7
fear avoidance 116, 184
fentanyl 92

G

gabapentin 95, 122, 176, 178
gastrointestinal function 80
gastrointestinal ulceration 89
gate control theory 5, 10–12, 17–20,
    165
gender 38, 117
genetics 22, 116, 173, 182
global policies 71–2
guided imagery 132
guidelines 78, 162, 180

H

headache 114, 131
heat therapy 129
herbs 133
heroin 92, 190
hyperalgesia 13, 21 (*see also* wind-up)
    primary hyperalgesia 13
hypochondiasis 185
hypnosis 131–2

I

ibuprofen 88
improving practice 59–63
immune response 22
immune suppression 79
implantable devices 124
incapacity benefit 193–4
information-giving 20, 85, 103–4
initial health assessment 29
injections 66

institutional policies 43, 67, 69–70
itch 92, 94
isolation 136

J

job satisfaction 195
journal group 157

K

kappa receptor 15–16, 92, 93
ketamine 95, 123, 176, 179
knowledge 56–9, 86, 95, 119

L

laxatives 99
learning disabilities 155–6
Leeds Assessment of Neuropathic
    Symptoms and Signs (LANSS) 38,
    41–2
leukotrienes 13–14
lignocaine 123, 178
limbic system 22, 130
litigation 194
local anaesthetic 21, 102–3, 123, 176
locus of control 20, 29
London Hospital pain observation chart
    36
low back pain 108, 128
low expectation about pain relief 65, 78

M

malingering 192
manipulation 128
massage 104, 127–8
McGill Pain Questionnaire (*see* Short-
    form)
methadone 93
mexilitine 123, 178
mind–body approaches 126–30
monoamine oxidase inhibitors 93
mood disorder 183–7
morphine 15, 87, 90, 91, 122, 162
mu receptor 15–16, 92, 93
Munchausen syndrome 186
multimodal 85, 89, 98, 182

muscle
  relaxants 123
  spasm 122
  tension 104, 131
music therapy 105, 133
misconceptions 57–8, 65, 96, 155, 187

N

nalbuphine 93
naloxone 16, 94
national policies 70–1
neonates and preverbal children 34, 156–64
  assessment guidelines 162
  non-pharmacological strategies 163
  pharmacological strategies 162
nerve block 7, 85, 103
  regional 124–5
  hip block 152
neuromatrix theory 21–2, 165
neuropathic pain 90, 114, 122, 125, 178
neurosignature 22
nitrous oxide 97–8
NMC code of conduct 126
n-methyl-D-aspartate acid (NMDA) 21, 93, 95, 123
nociceptive pain 178
nociceptors 6–12
non-pharmacological approaches 103–7, 125–36
non-steroidal anti-inflammatory drugs (NSAIDs) 13–14, 87–9, 122–3, 162, 176, 178
  topical 88, 98
norpethidine 93
NSAID *see* non-steroidal anti-inflammatory drugs
numbers needed to treat (NNT) 87
numerical scales 35–6
nurse prescribing 70, 71
  independent 71
  supplementary 71
nursing homes 146
nutritional supplements 134

O

oedema 122
older person 4, 146–54
  cognitively impaired 149–54
  common causes of pain 148
  observable indicators of pain 150
opioid 7, 8, 14–16, 21, 27, 98, 99, 102, 123, 124, 178, 179, 182, 188
  induced itch 92, 94
  intravenous 84
  receptors 7, 14–17, 89
  side effects 16, 83
  use 89–94
  weaker opioids 89–90
opium poppy 15, 89, 91
organisational aspects 67
osteoporosis 123
oxycodone 92

P

pain
  behaviour 149–52, 156–60
  belief in 118, 136
  cancer 4, 96
  central 178
  chemicals 6, 13–16
  consequences 3–4, 79–80
  definitions 4–6, 113, 114
  diaries 43, 153
  following day case surgery 3
  generators 114–17
  implications 66–7
  incident 30, 92
  inflicted 79
  in the community 3
  in hospital 3
  modulation 12–16
  neuropathic 90, 114, 122, 125, 178
  nociceptive 178
  perception 12, 16–17
  physical signs 31
  physical techniques for managing pain 126–30
  plasticity 17, 21, 116
  postoperative 3, 27, 77
paracetamol 86–7

Parkinson's disease 114
patch technology 124
patient barriers to effective pain
    management 63–7
patient-controlled analgesia (PCA) 46,
    85, 101–2, 191
patient group directives 70
patients' perspectives 78–80, 117–19
PCA see patient-controlled analgesia
personality 116
pethidine 93
phantom limb pain 22, 103
pharmacist 81
pharmacological approaches 86–95,
    120–5
phenytoin 122
physical dependence 188
physical techniques for managing pain
    126–30
physiotherapist 81
phytodolor 133
placebo 134–5
platelet
    adhesiveness 14, 79
    aggregation 88
    function 87
pneumothorax 98, 127
postherpetic neuralgia 116
postoperative nausea and vomiting 80,
    127
post-traumatic stress disorder 185
pre-emptive analgesia 21
pregabalin 122
professional collaboration 136–7 (see also
    teamwork)
prostaglandins 13, 87
protocol development 70
pseudo-addictive behaviours 192
psychogenic pain 173
psychological interventions 130–3,
    175–7
psychosocial factors 116, 192
pulmonary embolism 79

Q

quality improvement 62
quality of life 80, 113, 179, 196

R

radiotherapy 123
reflexology 130
relaxation 85, 104–5, 131, 163
relief from responsibility 195
religion (see culture)
renal colic 93
renal failure 103
renal function 14, 92, 93
respiratory depression 16, 96
respiratory function 79
Reye's syndrome 88
rheumatoid arthritis 114
Royal Colleges report 80

S

sea bands 127
secondary gain/loss 192–7
second pain 8
sedation 92, 96, 101, 122
self-efficacy 116
self-esteem 136, 192
sensitisation 13
sensory-discriminative dimension 17,
    19, 22
serotonin 127
Short-form McGill Pain Questionnaire
    37–8
sickle-cell disease 180–3
    guide to management 183
single nurse administration of drugs
    69–70
skilled companionship 105–6
sleep disturbance 80
snoezelen 136, 176, 177
social activities 136, 192
social policy 193–4
somatoform disorder 185–6
spinal cord stimulation 128
spinal injury 177–80
    mechanisms 178
standards 67, 71, 80
    JCAHO 43
stereotyping 165–6
steroids 122–3
sticky labels 70, 82–3, 161

stress 20, 22, 103, 116, 173, 185, 195
substance misuse 187–92
   symptoms 188–9
   management 189–91
   pseudo-addiction 192
substance P 13–14, 123
substantia gelatinosa 8, 12
suffering 22–3

T

teamwork 59, 70, 189 (*see also* professional collaboration)
TENS *see* transcutaneous electrical nerve stimulation
tolerance 96, 182, 188, 189
touch 9
tramadol 90
transcutaneous electrical nerve stimulation (TENS) 107, 128, 179
trigeminal neuralgia 122

trusting therapeutic relationship 135–6

U

urinary retention 94

V

verbal communication 29–30
visual analogue scale 35
visual displays of pain 30

W

willow bark 133
wind-up 21, 123 (*see also* hyperalgesia)
withdrawal 188–9
Wisconsin Policy Unit 71
work
   demands 34, 68
   environment 58
World Health Organization 4, 72, 98, 99